LOW BLOOD SUGAR
(Hypoglycaemia)

The 20th Century Epidemic?

by

MARTIN BUDD
N.D., D.O., Lic.Ac.

Sterling Publishing Co., Inc. New York

Library of Congress Cataloging in Publication Data

Budd, Martin.
  Low blood sugar (hypoglycaemia)

  Includes bibliographical references and index.
  1. Hypoglycemia. I. Title.
RC662.2.B83 1983   616.3'998   83-5053
ISBN 0-8069-7792-2 (pbk.)

Previously 0-7225-0589-2

Low Blood Sugar

Explains what hypoglycaemia (low blood sugar) is and how it is often the root cause of many other ailments such as fatigue, depression, headaches and neurotic behaviour; and looks at the causes, symptoms, diagnosis and treatment of this misunderstood problem. Includes case histories.

CONTENTS

INTRODUCTION

Why is low blood sugar a common problem when many people eat far too much sugar? Why do sufferers from high blood sugar (diabetes or hyperglycaemia) and low blood sugar (hypoglycaemia) have to follow similar diets when their problems seem to be opposite? (N.B. The terms 'hypo' and 'hyper' which recur throughout the text mean 'too little' and 'too much', respectively.) Is sugar good for us or harmful, and does it really matter whether the sugar we eat is brown or white? How can sugar affect our memory and concentration and even our personalities? Are honey and molasses also sugars or harmless natural substitutes? What is the connection between low blood sugar and such diverse complaints as alcoholism, migraine, asthma, depression, arthritis, obesity and epilepsy? What is the relationship between sugar and fat, and does sugar really provide all our energy needs? What is the difference between reactive hypoglycaemia, functional hypoglycaemia and relative hypoglycaemia?

When discussing hypoglycaemia with patients, or when lecturing, I have frequently been asked similar questions, perhaps because hypoglycaemia is a confusing, complex and contradictory disease. In this book, I set out to answer these and other questions.

Although officially 'discovered' in 1924 by Seale Harris, an American physician, the medical establishment insists that hypoglycaemia is an extremely rare condition and that the functional hypoglycaemia due to faulty diet is a trendy condition invented by health-food faddists. Some nutritionists and scientists claim that hypoglycaemia is a temporary, easily-rectified imbalance; others see it as the basis of many serious diseases, a contributing factor to cancer, heart disease, diabetes, asthma and arthritis, etc.

Definitions of hypoglycaemia range from 'the opposite of diabetes' (hyperinsulinism) to the less simplistic view that blood sugar deficiency is due to complex interactions between the glandular, nervous and digestive systems. Even the diagnosis of hypoglycaemia is a subject of controversy. Many practitioners feel that a six-hour glucose tolerance test is a satisfactory and conclusive method of diagnosing hypoglycaemia. Others consider the test to be misleading and ambiguous and prefer to base their diagnosis on careful assessments of the patient's history and symptoms.

Perhaps you can begin to understand why I consider hypoglycaemia to be confusing and contradictory. It is perhaps unfortunate that the major symptoms of hypoglycaemia, e.g. fatigue, depression, headache and neurotic behaviour, are often diagnosed as being due to stress. Even in the second half of the twentieth century most doctors insist on the separation of disorders of the mind and body. It may well be that hypoglycaemia is the bridge which links many mental and physical symptoms, and that correct nutrition is the key to both.

1
SYMPTOMS OF HYPOGLYCAEMIA

Hypoglycaemia means literally low (hypo) blood sugar (glycaemia), or an abnormally low level of glucose in the blood. This definition is deceptively simple for it is possible to have symptoms of low blood sugar with a *normal* level of sugar in the blood. Quite obviously the actual level of blood sugar is, by itself, an insufficient basis for the diagnosis of hypoglycaemia. This paradox will be explained later in the book in Chapter 10, on diagnosis. Another problem with the diagnosis of hypoglycaemia is that almost all the symptoms of hypoglycaemia can be caused by other pathological conditions.

General Indications
To discuss the diversity of symptoms caused by low blood sugar would take up most of this book. The list below, however, is a representative selection of the most common symptoms:

Fatigue	Anxiety	Depression
Irritability	Forgetfulness	Poor concentration
Indigestion	Breathlessness	Panic feelings
Headaches	Migraine	Asthma
Overweight	Food cravings	Excessive smoking
Alcoholism	Vertigo	Sweating
Pre-menstrual tension	Muscular stiffness	Phobias
Numbness	Blurred vision	Cold extremities
Joint pain	Fainting and blackouts	Convulsions
Nightmares	Lack of sex drive	Allergies
Heart disease	Angina	Suicidal tendencies
Epilepsy	Stomach cramps	Stomach ulcers
Hyperactivity		

I am sure there will be many eyebrows raised at the great variety and number of symptoms mentioned and, at first sight, it is difficult to imagine that there is a common theme to all these conditions. (All this could be a hypochondriac's dream come true! He can tell his friends with a certain pride that he has hypoglycaemia and wait for the murmurings of sympathy.) Interestingly enough, many of the symptoms of low blood sugar are classed by doctors as 'stress disorders' and I hope to show, by describing the effect of sugar on the nervous system, that many of these symptoms are in fact due to nutritional imbalances and not personality failings. You may also see several of your own symptoms on the list; but simply to scan this list, recognize one's own symptoms and diagnose low blood sugar is clearly not the answer. As previously stated, many of these symptoms may have other causes, not least of which *could* be stress. It is therefore essential, in order to accurately diagnose hypoglycaemia, that more objective diagnostic methods be used. These include detailed case history taking and the six-hour glucose tolerance test.

At some time in their lives most people experience one or more of these symptoms. This is usually due to transient hypoglycaemia, which is defined as a temporary or passing drop in blood sugar level, and this is soon rectified by the body's own sugar regulation mechanism. Once a balance is achieved, the symptoms usually disappear. If, however, there is a real long-term imbalance in the sugar regulation the symptoms may well disappear or change, but they will always return unless the actual imbalance is corrected.

Now let us look more closely at the way in which a drop in the blood sugar directly affects the various organs and systems of the body, giving rise to the symptoms listed above. In this way you will begin to understand why the blood sugar level is so important to the normal running of the body. The effects can be classified as follows.

Nervous System Changes

The main nutrient needed by the nervous system is glucose. There is no really adequate substitute and, although other substances are involved, they cannot replace glucose. Unfortunately, it is not fully understood just how glucose acts on the nervous system, but it has been noted that when a healthy patient is injected with insulin (the opposite of glucose), there occurs, within minutes, profound and sudden changes in the efficiency of the nervous system. This is completely reversed by an injection of glucose. This tends to confirm that the nervous system requires a continuous supply of glucose in order to function efficiently.

Although the weight of an adult brain is only 2 per cent of the total body weight, the activity of the brain, in terms of utilization of glucose, may amount to 20-25 per cent of the total body activity. In spite of this, the total amount of glucose concentrated within the brain, at any one time, would under normal conditions, be exhausted in ten to fifteen minutes. The actual effects of glucose starvation on the brain and nerve tissue are as follows:

1. Insufficient oxygen.

2. Reduction in specific substances within the brain that are essential for nervous activity.

Circulatory Changes

Not surprisingly the system first affected by a drop in the blood sugar level is the circulatory system. This, of course, includes the heart and blood vessels. When the blood sugar drops, the body automatically reacts in an attempt to restore balance to the system. The main changes that occur involve the adrenal gland, part of which is concerned with the body's reaction to stress situations. This means that if a person has persistent low blood sugar, he may have symptoms similar to those produced by chronic stress. These can include:

1. An irregular increase in the heart rate causing palpitations and breathing difficulties.

2. Angina-like symptoms involving reduction in circulation to the heart muscle, chest cramp and pain in the chest and arms.

3. A general withdrawal of blood to deal with the 'stress effects', causing coldness of the hands and feet, muscular cramp and a poor adaptation to temperature changes.

Glandular Changes

The changes involved in the glandular system following a drop in the blood glucose level are widespread and could well provide sufficient material for another book. It may, however, be of interest simply to list the glands affected, to emphasize the wide influence of blood sugar imbalance.

1. Pituitary gland. This is the master control gland influencing the thyroid and adrenal glands.

2. Adrenal glands. These glands produce adrenalin and cortisone. It is the persistent stimulation of these glands in a patient suffering from hypoglycaemia that provides the link between hypoglycaemia and rheumatoid arthritis, as overactivity of part of the adrenal glands can cause reduction in the availability of cortisone which gives some protection against joint injury and inflammation.

3. Thyroid gland. Changes that occur with thyroid activity are of less significance than the other glands although, like the adrenal and pituitary glands, the thyroid secretions are essentially antagonistic to insulin, and thyroid imbalance may contribute to a blood sugar imbalance.

Digestive Changes

The changes in gastric (stomach) activity are mainly due to the increased insulin level in the blood that occurs with hypoglycaemia rather than the actual deficiency of glucose. A standard hospital test to assess the efficiency of digestive activity is to administer to the patient an injection of insulin. This prompts a rapid and predictable increase in the amount of stomach acids which are then measured. It follows that if this test has such an effect, the fluctuations of the insulin level in the blood, as in hypoglycaemia, would have a similar effect. Indeed, in practice, I find that many patients suffering from stomach ulcers, heartburn, hiatus hernia and other digestive ailments, very often have an underlying blood sugar imbalance.

Psychological Changes

After discussing the effects of low blood sugar on the brain and nervous system it is not surprising to learn that a patient suffering from hypoglycaemia may also have personality problems. The most common symptoms involving the low blood sugar patient are depression, anxiety and mental confusion. Many researchers, particularly in the United States, consider that hypoglycaemia is the main contributing factor to such serious personality problems as schizophrenia and paranoia. We know that hypoglycaemia affects the adrenal glands and that the adrenal glands are the body's main defence mechanism against stress. It therefore seems likely that the hypoglycaemic patient becomes involved in a vicious circle of adrenal exhaustion causing anxiety and the anxiety causing further exhaustion and stress. Unfortunately, most people suffering from stress tend to overeat, or eat all the wrong foods or miss meals altogether, thus aggravating further the blood sugar imbalance.

Miscellaneous Effects

It is an interesting fact that diabetic patients rarely have asthma. In fact, there are very few cases on record of a true asthma patient having diabetes; the main exception is the condition known as cardiac asthma. Many asthma patients find to their delight in their late 40's and 50's that their asthma symptoms subside. The reason for this is that they often become pre-diabetic; their blood sugar has become raised above normal level thus protecting them from asthma.

The key to this enigma is a substance called histamine. This substance is naturally present in the body and has a variety of uses, not least is its role in controlling osmosis (passage of water) between the body membranes. It is well known that, if the histamine level increases, the characteristic symptoms are hay fever, skin rashes and asthma. The link between histamine and the blood sugar is that histamine and glucose are on separate ends of a see-saw. If the glucose level drops the histamine level rises and vice versa. It follows that a patient who has low blood sugar may, under certain conditions, also have asthma or hay fever and, indeed, many hypoglycaemic patients have children with hay fever. It should be said that low blood sugar is not the *only* cause of asthma; there are certain types of asthma due entirely to stress or extreme sensitivity to various allergens.

The other system of the body affected by hypoglycaemia is the musculo-skeletal system, in other words, muscles and joints. As already explained, the effect of the adrenal glands and, in particular, cortisone on joint injury and inflammation is well documented, hence the apparently miraculous symptom relief afforded to rheumatoid arthritis patients when cortisone is taken or injected. If the adrenal glands' efficiency is overworked or impaired owing to prolonged low blood sugar, it seems entirely possible that the hypoglycaemic patient would be prone to arthritis and similar problems.

2

THE HYPOGLYCAEMIC
PERSONALITY

It is customary to attribute the growth and development of personality to a combination of inherited tendencies and environmental influences. The 'inheritance' school maintain that personality and intelligence are shaped by the genetically laid down characteristics of race and body-type, our personality being determined at birth by these influences. The 'environmental' school believe that we are virtually born with a blank mind which is influenced and moulded in terms of personality and intelligence by our environment. These environmental influences include social class, education, economic considerations, domestic pressures, occupation and health.

Although the controversy over these two fundamental causes of personality has dominated much of the thinking of psychologists, educationists and other workers, recent attitudes support the more balanced view that personality and intelligence are shaped by a combination of both influences.

Leaving aside for the present the question of intelligence, most of us have a many-faceted personality. Our education, parental guidance, choice of partner, employment and religion are all likely to act on our moods, attitudes and beliefs to make us the people we are. A popularly held view is that our adult personality, as presented to the world, is unchanging and unchangeable. We recognize and accept that some people are bad-tempered, moody or depressed, while others are gentle, care-free and optimistic. If someone we know is always angry and aggressive, we usually accept that 'this is the way he is'.

Physical States and Personality
Many destructive or negative emotions and attitudes are linked with physical symptoms, e.g. depression with fatigue,

fear with palpitations and coldness. Physical illnesses associated with stressful attitudes or emotions are often termed 'psycho-somatic disorders' or simply 'mind and body illness'. The medical view is that stress produces a physical effect and the treatment of such a disorder needs to be directed at alleviating or masking the stress. This is attempted by prescribing a variety of drugs or by the use of various psychotherapeutic procedures, e.g. psycho-analysis.

The psychologist, William James, noted in the last century that every emotion has its physical counterpart. This observation appears to support the view that stress affects the physical body, and only by removing the stress can the physical symptom be relieved (i.e. stress-induced stomach ulcers, stress-induced eczema). However, this sequence of cause and effect can be reversed according to the 'chicken and egg principle' – which comes first, the faulty emotion behind the stress, or the physical symptom accompanying the stress?

In practice I have observed that the majority of stressful personalities have accompanying physical symptoms. These physical symptoms often *precede* the emotional changes, e.g. depression preceded by fatigue; anxiety preceded by headache, palpitations and dizziness; agoraphobia preceded by feelings of panic; suicidal tendencies preceded by menstrual disorders and exhaustion.

As explained in the previous chapter, optimum nutrition to the nervous system is a prerequisite of normal health. If the supply of glucose to the nerve cells is deficient, physical symptoms and actual personality changes may occur. The personality of the person suffering from low blood sugar can alter to such an extent that, to all intents and purposes, he or she becomes a different person. Moreover, patients with hypoglycaemia tend to share the same personality patterns.

Before examining the available evidence to support the concept of a hypoglycaemic personality, it may be of value to define more fully the characteristics of a typical hypoglycaemic sufferer, and appreciate the difficulties in diagnosing hypo-glycaemia without laboratory evidence.

Difficulties of Diagnosis
The level of glucose in our blood is constantly fluctuating, for demands are made on available glucose when exercising, under stress, during pregnancy and prior to menstruation. In

each case there is a tendency for the glucose level to reduce whilst, not surprisingly, our food and drink has the opposite effect of increasing the glucose level. Even the time of day may be significant as the glucose level reduces between meals and at night, or whenever food is avoided for more than three hours.

Diabetic patients on insulin are only too well aware of the sensitive nature of glucose balance as they are obliged to control and monitor constantly their activities and food, as well as their insulin requirements. Most of us, however, are blissfully unaware of the importance of the blood glucose level and the dramatic symptoms that can develop when the level is reduced.

The lowering of blood glucose and the subsequent reduction in available glucose to the nervous system leads to a variety of symptoms as already outlined. Unfortunately for the patient and the diagnostician, the symptoms are neither constant nor predictable, as the available glucose varies to such an extent that sudden and severe physical and emotional symptoms can develop within fifteen to twenty minutes following a drop in the glucose level. When the glucose level normalizes ('normal' being the optimum level for that patient) the changes in mood, sudden coldness, palpitations, sweating and many other symptoms attributed to hypoglycaemia, rapidly recede. These sudden shifts in mood and symptoms are often diagnosed as stress-induced. In other words, the patient seeing his doctor with the typical symptoms of low blood sugar is often classified as a neurotic, anxious personality. Regrettably such a diagnosis, with the possible prescription of antidepressants or sedatives, only creates more confusion and worry for the patient. This additional worry can lead to a further imbalance in the blood sugar level and produce an aggravation of the hypoglycaemic symptoms. Hence a vicious circle is achieved.

This train of events is not always so straightforward as Figure 1 suggests, for there is often genuine stress in addition to the hypoglycaemia due to other causes, and this obviously complicates the picture. The fact remains, however, that hypoglycaemia alone can cause the symptoms of stress and a hypoglycaemic personality is very vulnerable to additional stress, often being quite unable to deal with even day-to-day problems. The anxiety created in the patient's mind by a diagnosis of 'nerves' is more damaging if the patient knows full

Figure 1. Diagram showing the relation between hypoglycaemia
       and stress.

well that he is not under stress and indeed has nothing to
worry about. I often hear the comment from patients that they
cannot understand why they feel so tense and anxious as they
have a settled and happy life with no worries. The medical
explanation for anxiety without cause is to suggest that the
symptoms, in some strange way, arise from within the patient.
This is termed 'endogenous' and is treated as a psychiatric
problem with psychotherapy or drugs. It is of great relief to the
patient who feels he is 'going mad', or states that he is 'unable
to cope any more', to be told that there is not a nervous
breakdown round the corner, nor is his personality breaking
up owing to some hidden subconscious mental conflict. What
is happening is probably due to an imbalance in his metabolism
involving an insufficient supply of fuel to the nervous system
(i.e. low blood sugar) which in the majority of cases is easy to
treat and often completely reversible.

The Evidence

Having stated that an apparently simple commonplace occurrence involving a drop in the blood glucose level can give rise to profound and sudden physical and emotional symptoms, I feel obliged to justify my comments with a little supportive evidence. Researchers in many countries have, over the last fifty years, examined the problem of hypoglycaemia and the conclusions fall into two distinctly opposing camps. There are those who state that a certain type of personality may give rise to hypoglycaemia, whilst others maintain that hypoglycaemia produces a typical, well-defined personality. The evidence in favour of the latter view is, however, overwhelming. Especially when one appreciates that hypoglycaemia resulting from stomach surgery or insulin therapy can also give rise to the characteristic hypoglycaemic personality.

In the early 1920's Dr Banting and his co-workers (the discoverers of insulin) observed that hypoglycaemia caused by insulin overdose produced symptoms of hunger, weakness and anxiety. These unpleasant symptoms, with which diabetics are usually familiar, are not produced by the insulin itself but by the sudden slump in the level of glucose in the blood, termed a 'hypo' effect. In 1933 two American physicians, Graham and Womack, stated that, 'It is important to emphasize that in many cases the neurological and psychiatric aspects of the condition are so prominent that many of the patients with chronic hypoglycaemia have been referred primarily to neurologists and psychiatrists for treatment'.[1]

Seale Harris, acknowledged as the discoverer of hypoglycaemia, also noted that patients with hypoglycaemia symptoms are often misdiagnosed as neurotic or psychiatric cases. He considered that emotional symptoms can be caused by organic malfunction and reported that dietary treatment resulted in the relief of the symptoms.[2]

Fabrykant, an authority on hypoglycaemia, stated in 1953 that 'personality disorders were secondary to biochemical changes'.[3] In a detailed examination of hypoglycaemia and personality Dr Anthony and his co-workers concluded that their results supported the association of hypoglycaemia with personality disorders. They found that 27 from 31 selected hypoglycaemia patients showed abnormal personality profiles when subjected to standardized psychological testing. Furthermore, three of the remaining four patients were borderline.

Their conclusions were summarized as follows:

1. Patients with hypoglycaemia of varying aetiology (diabetic, alimentary or idiopathic) all show the same personality pattern suggesting that hypoglycaemia causes personality disorder.

2. Low blood glucose values with counter-regulatory endocrine reactions constitute a plausible organic explanation for the peculiar mental symptoms that trouble these patients. Our data indicate that reactive hypoglycaemia is almost invariably accompanied by significant personality disorder.[4]

The British Medical Journal, 20 April, 1974, carried an article which stated, 'The finding that patients with hypoglycaemia of varying aetiology showed the same personality pattern supports the view that hypoglycaemia causes the abnormality of personality'.[5]

In hypoglycaemia the nervous system is deprived of essential fuel (i.e. glucose) and the brain is subsequently affected. Changes of mood, depression, anxiety, irritability, poor concentration, feelings of panic and suicidal tendencies are just a few of the symptoms that can be produced by this so often misdiagnosed problem. Recent research in the U.S. suggests that even psychiatric and schizoid tendencies may, in part, be due to low blood sugar.

Two researchers, Dr W Beebe and Dr O Wendell, wrote in a paper on psychiatric patients that, 'Of those patients categorized as chronic schizophrenics 70 per cent exhibited some form of hypoglycaemia'.[6]

Dr R Meiers wrote in his paper 'Relative Hypoglycaemia in Schizophrenia', 'Relative Hypoglycaemia is present in up to 70 per cent of patients with schizophrenia. Inadequate diet exists in almost 100 per cent. Since the diet used in the treatment of relative hypoglycaemia also improved nutrition in general, it is a valuable adjunct in the treatment of all patients with schizophrenia'.[7]

In Chapter 12 I will provide case histories to illustrate the hypoglycaemic personality and, I hope to show the link between physical cause and emotional effect. Hypoglycaemia is not the only cause of disordered personalities, yet it may well be the commonest *physical* cause and certainly the most frequently misdiagnosed.

3

DISCOVERY AND CAUSES

Discovery

Medical discoveries are often made by chance rather than by painstaking research and analysis. One open door may lead to others, for much in nature and science is connected. One clue leads to another, like a treasure trail, and one proven hypothesis may open up a whole field of related study. In this way, the chance observations of an obscure American doctor more than half a century ago led to the discovery that reactive hypoglycaemia is an important cause of a great variety of symptoms. Seale Harris was a general practitioner living in the state of Alabama and a contemporary of Banting and Best, the co-discoverers of the role of insulin in diabetes.

Harris noticed that many diabetic patients attending the new insulin clinics developed symptoms of *low* blood sugar. This paradox is not difficult to understand if you see insulin and sugar as being on opposite ends of the scale. When there is balance the scale is level, but if one is in excess, the other is deficient. Many diabetics have difficulty in accurately judging their insulin requirements and often overdose themselves, producing a condition known as hyperinsulinism which consequently causes hypoglycaemia. This 'hypo' or insulin effect is characterized by symptoms of anxiety, fatigue, breathlessness and palpitations. Essentially the diabetic has swung from high to low blood sugar due to an inappropriate increase in the blood insulin level. Fortunately, this is a transient effect. Most diabetics learn to avoid the 'hypo' situation by carefully balancing their insulin dosage, diet and energy output; at the same time regularly monitoring their blood and urine sugar levels.

To return to Dr Harris, he noted that he had in his practice several patients who exhibited symptoms of the 'hypo' reaction on a regular basis, but who were *not* diabetic and who were, therefore, not taking insulin. He accurately concluded that these patients probably experienced the unpleasant symptoms of hypoglycaemia as a result of overactivity or imbalance in their insulin-producing apparatus. This complex mechanism involves the islet glands of the pancreas, the liver, to some extent the pituitary, thyroid and adrenal glands and many other factors which play their part in sugar metabolism.

In 1924 Seale Harris presented his theories in a paper published in the *Journal of the American Medical Association*.[8] His reasoning on the possible causes of hypoglycaemia in non-diabetic patients led him to conclude that many glands of the body can be 'hypo' or 'hyper' active and that frequently underactivity (hypo) is preceded by overactivity (hyper). This concept is not difficult to appreciate as overactivity, with subsequent exhaustion or damage, is a characteristic of many organs and systems within the body. Any overworked machine usually malfunctions.

Dr Harris discussed his ideas with Dr Banting who agreed that the role of insulin in hypoglycaemia offered a new aspect to the study of blood sugar balance, presenting a mirror image to the diabetic situation. No papers on this topic had appeared in medical literature prior to Seale Harris's historic work, but his discoveries led to a glut of similar papers in journals all over the world.

The American *Annals of Internal Medicine* (1936) included a further paper by Harris.[2] This definitive statement precisely classified the causes and symptoms of hypoglycaemia. Although subsequent research has shown that the relationship of low blood sugar to excess insulin in the blood is not so simplistic as defined by Harris, it is now recognized that the whole glandular system is involved in the blood sugar balance.

Causes
Having outlined the events that led to the discovery of reactive hypoglycaemia, it is important to discuss the main groups of causes.

1. *Delayed insulin secretion.* Delay, as in early diabetes, causes an inappropriate elevation of insulin at a time when blood glucose is falling.

2. *Alimentary or surgical.* Symptoms known as the 'dumping syndrome' – this involves a rapid emptying of the stomach contents allowing rapid absorption of glucose and resulting reactive hypoglycaemia. This can occur anything from one to four hours after eating.

3. *Nervous factors.* Possible vagal overactivity and stress situations leading to adrenal exhaustion and thyrotoxicosis, etc.

4. *Insulin antagonists.* Suppression of secretion of contra-insulin agents, chiefly growth hormone, adrenal and pituitary secretions. Treatment by cortisol and growth hormone bring about rapid improvement.

5. *The Unknown 90 per cent.* These are mainly thought to be idiopathic, hereditary and largely nutritional in origin, the chief influence being an inherited characteristic coupled with a high starch diet; this gradually gives rise to excessive insulin production.

Perhaps in the fifth cause mentioned the word 'Unknown' should be in inverted commas as in my own practice I find that the majority of patients suffering from reactive hypoglycaemia have a characteristic pattern of inherited influences and faulty diet. The typical hypoglycaemic make-up will be discussed in the chapter on diagnosis, for this book is mainly concerned with reactive hypoglycaemia caused by the 'unknown 90 per cent'. I should explain that the medical establishment is not in agreement with the concept of low blood sugar as a 'disease entity' (a condition producing symptoms). Hypoglycaemia is generally seen as a common symptom associated with many disorders. Yet, according to many American nutritionists and non-medical practitioners in Europe, reactive hypoglycaemia is recognized as a condition produced by a variety of causes and giving rise to a large range of clearly-defined symptoms. This is usually caused by the combinations of influences detailed below. It may seem rather illogical to deal with causes after discussing symptoms in Chapter 1, but I believe readers can relate more immediately to symptoms than to causes.

Hereditary Factors

Although we all recognize that characteristics pass through generations, e.g. posture, personality, poor teeth, premature baldness, chest and heart problems, etc., there are, in fact, very few inherited diseases. The list includes syphilis, diabetes and haemophilia. Although other diseases that are directly inherited are more obscure and include certain rare blood disorders and musculo-skeletal problems (chorea and ataxia, etc.) there are, however, many conditions that can be traced through families that have a common theme, i.e. blood sugar imbalance.

If you refer to the list of symptoms of hypoglycaemia in Chapter 1 you will note the following conditions that often run through several generations of the same family – diabetes, epilepsy, asthma, hay fever, migraine, depression, obesity, rheumatoid arthritis. The diabetic patient may produce a diabetic child as the pancreatic deficiency is directly inherited. Paradoxically, the child of a diabetic patient may be born with a normal pancreas that is simply oversensitive rather than deficient and this sensitivity may lead to an eventual over-activity as a result of faulty diet which, in turn, may lead to hyperinsulinism and reactive hypoglycaemia. In my own practice we always enquire about family health, of parents and grandparents and of children and grandchildren.

Table 1 shows the characteristic low blood sugar conditions that run through families. Patients are always asked for details of family health including diabetes, asthma, hay fever and migraine. The list is composed of fifty patients selected from my practice who were diagnosed as hypoglycaemic. They were chosen in strict sequence to avoid giving a biased result.

Organic and Reactive Hypoglycaemia

Some American doctors who specialize in the diagnosis and treatment of hypoglycaemia maintain that we all suffer from the symptoms of hypoglycaemia at some time in our lives. Some of us, however, are more sensitive to sugar than others. It should be stated that the Western diet contributes to hypoglycaemia owing to the refining, concentrating and high pressure marketing of starch and sugar products.

There are many different causes for hypoglycaemia, including pancreatic tumours, pancreatitis, gastric surgery, adrenal tumours, glandular diseases, etc. However, I am discussing the commonest type of hypoglycaemia known as

Table 1. Chart Showing Hypoglycaemic Conditions in the
Families of 50 Patients with Reactive Hypoglycaemia

Patient's Condition	Grandparents	Mother	Father	Children	Siblings
M		D			
M		H			
St		A			
M	D				
M	A				A
H & F		M	D		A
M			M		
M		A & M			A
M					HF
F					A
O		D	A		
F		M		A	
F		M	D		M
F		M			
M				M	A
A	A				
B				A	M
M		M			M
M		M	A		
F					A
St	D				
M		A			
O		M			A
M		M		A	
M					A
H		D	M	M	
F		D			
M			D		
M		M			M
B	M				
M		M	M		M
De		M			
H	M				E
F	D		H		
M		M			
M		M			A
A					A

For Key see overleaf ...

Table 1 continued

Patient's Condition	Grandparents	Mother	Father	Children	Siblings
M			H		
H					A
E					A
M	D				
De			De		HF
De					
HF					HF
M				HF	A
E					M
M			A		
De		M		HF	M
M	A	M		M	
F	A	M			

Key

A	– Asthma		H	– Headaches
B	– Blackouts or dizziness		HF	– Hay fever
D	– Diabetes		M	– Migraine
De	– Depression or anxiety		O	– Obesity
E	– Epilepsy		St	– Stomach Disorders
F	– Fatigue			

reactive hypoglycaemia (also called functional hypoglycaemia and relative hypoglycaemia).

The main difference between organic hypoglycaemia and reactive hypoglycaemia lies in the fasting glucose levels. Where there is organic disease causing hypoglycaemia, the glucose fasting level is invariably low. In reactive hypoglycaemia the fasting level of glucose may be normal or even a little above normal, and the body over-reacts to glucose by producing an excess of insulin which creates the drop in blood glucose. In hypoglycaemia due to functional disease the symptoms are usually continuous, while in reactive hypoglycaemia the symptoms fluctuate according to type of food, time of day, etc. An inappropriate and unnecessary high sugar diet causes a situation where the blood is flooded with glucose it cannot use. Although some may be stored as glycogen and deposited in the liver or muscles, the balance leads to an over-reaction by the insulin apparatus. In this way the body is conditioned over a period of years to produce more and more insulin until the time is reached where the slightest increase in blood glucose causes a sudden and dramatic increase in the blood insulin.

The final link in this chain of events is the role of the adrenal glands. As the blood sugar drops, the glands produce adrenalin and cortisone to facilitate the release of stored glucose. In this way, further stress symptoms – so characteristic of hypoglycaemia – are produced and the circle starts again.

It has been said that the hypoglycaemia patient of today is the diabetic of tomorrow. As we are talking about totally opposite conditions, this may be at first difficult to understand. Hypoglycaemia, as we know, is characterized by a conditioned over-reaction of the insulin production causing low blood sugar. If, at around sixty years old, the patient's overworked pancreas finally gives up and becomes exhausted, the pendulum swings the other way and the production of insulin is insufficient, thus leading to diabetes.

The diets for hypoglycaemia and diabetes are remarkably similar. The low blood sugar patient avoids sugar to allow the pancreas to reduce and normalize insulin output, while the diabetic needs to avoid sugar because his body does not produce enough insulin to convert, transport and utilize the sugar. In many glandular imbalances, whether affecting thyroid, pituitary or adrenal glands, the line between overactivity and underactivity may be very finely drawn, as an imbalance can occur either way, but in the early stages the problem can often be reversed if correct treatment is applied.

4
SUGAR:
AN UNNATURAL HISTORY

To most people sugar is the white or brown substance with which they sweeten tea or coffee. This is known as sucrose and is extracted from beet or cane. The other main sugars consumed are lactose (milk sugar) and fructose (fruit sugar). The whole sugar family, known as carbohydrates, is shown below. They are classified according to their complexity, the simple sugars being monosaccharides and the most complex sugars are polysaccharides consisting of many groups of simple units.

In studies it has been found that the average adult carbohydrate consumption can be broken down as follows:

Starch (bread, cereals, etc.)	50%
Sucrose (sugar)	35%
Lactose (milk, etc.)	7%
Glucose and fructose (fruit and vegetables)	8%

Early Use of Sugar

The general use of sugar probably began around 1000 B.C. in the later Bronze Age, the main source of sweetening for cereals and cooking being honey. At first wild bees' nests were ransacked but, with the spread of pastureland, crude beekeeping leading to hive manufacturing took place. The production of honey in the Bronze Age was secondary to the need for beeswax, an essential substance in the process of bronze casting. Understandably, people learned to enjoy the sweet flavour of the honey for it served as a seasoning as well as a sweetener. Although sugar was extracted from sugar cane in India several centuries before Christ, honey

Table 2. Classification of Carbohydrates (Simplified)

Mono-saccharides .... basic unit Di-saccharides .... 2 mono-saccharide units Poly-saccharides .... 10-10,000 mono-saccharide units
Mono-saccharides (single sugars): *Glucose (Dextrose):* Found in blood, oxidized in cells to provide energy. Stored in the liver as glycogen. *Fructose (Fruit sugar):* Found in fruit and honey – sweetest of the sugars. *Galactose:* Obtained from milk sugar, not found free in nature.
Di-saccharides (double sugars): *Sucrose (Cane or Beet sugar):* Not directly absorbed by blood stream, except after splitting by digestive enzymes in small intestine into the two single sugars glucose and fructose, which are then separately absorbed or converted to glycogen. *Maltose (Malt sugar):* Present in barley and in honey, though occurs chiefly as a result of starch breakdown by saliva and by secretions from the pancreas. Like sucrose it must be split by enzymes in the small intestine into glucose units before it can be used. *Lactose (Milk sugar):* Like the other di-saccharides, lactose cannot be utilized by the body until broken down by digestive enzymes into the two single sugars, glucose and galactose. In some infants a 'block' may exist whereby the galactose cannot be absorbed and the child will become ill, even fatally, unless milk is withheld.
Poly-saccharides: Examples are starch, dextrins, cellulose and glycogen. The poly-saccharides are made up of simple glucose units bonded together and cannot be utilized by the body until 'uncoupled' by digestive processes. They are insoluble in cold water, but cooking softens and ruptures cells and facilitates digestion.

remained the main sweetener, sugar being used chiefly as a medicine.

The Romans used honey exclusively in their cooking, and by Anglo-Saxon times honey was still the sweetening agent for food and drink. The production of honey became an essential part of country life, and laws controlling and taxing the ownership of hives were introduced.

After the Dark Ages following the fall of Rome, it was the Crusaders of the eleventh century who rediscovered honey in Europe. Also, the gradual spread of sugar cane production from India to Persia had been accelerated by the Arab conquests. As a result, cane was grown in North Africa and the Mediterranean isles by the tenth century. With the impetus of the Crusades, trade flourished between the Eastern Mediterranean and Europe and sugar became one of the most sought-after commodities.

Sugar at this time was very expensive, being rare and costly to import. It was only available to the very rich, and honey, being cheaper, was still the only sweetener for the poor. In medieval England sugar was regarded as a spice or flavouring, being used to flavour both sweet and savoury dishes. In the homes of the rich merchants and noblemen, even meat was dusted with sugar. It was also used as a medicine for a variety of ailments, particularly for convalescence and infections.

World Scale Production

With the colonizing of the many islands of the Americas in the fifteenth and sixteenth centuries, sugar cane was the ideal economic crop and was grown on an increasing scale. Barbados, Trinidad and Jamaica became part of the British Empire, while the Portuguese controlled the Azores, and the Spanish colonized the Canaries, Cuba and Puerto Rico. This led to an increase in the world production and consumption of sugar, and in the late sixteenth century there were fifty refineries in London alone.

In spite of the then heavy taxation on sugar importation, demand grew. In the reign of Elizabeth I, the consumption was 1 lb (450g) per person per year but, with the price equivalent in twentieth century prices of around £20 per lb, only the very wealthy could afford its regular use. Within a hundred years consumption rose to 4 lb (1.8 kg) per person and even the poorest folk bought a few ounces a week. It was still considered a good medicine and many prescriptions included sugar to purge the 'vapours' or 'melancholy'. The damaging effects of sugar were, however, beginning to be apparent: Elizabeth I had black teeth owing to her sugar craving.

Sugar consumption took a great surge upwards with the introduction of tea, coffee and chocolate in the eighteenth century. All these drinks are naturally slightly bitter, and tea with sugar became a favourite drink of the poor. By the late eighteenth century, sugar and tea were staple items in the inadequate diet of the poor in the industrial towns of England.

Present Consumption

This brings the story almost up to date, and the consumption of sugar has grown enormously in the last 150 years (see Figure 2).

As can be seen, we now eat 120 lb (54 kg) per year each. Obviously some eat more than others, yet most people, being confronted with these figures, will stoutly deny that they eat anywhere near the average of 2½ lb (1 kg) sugar a week. Much of the sugar we eat is not visible sugar: many items of food and drink contain sugar as a sweetener or preservative, and this 'hidden' sugar is included in the consumption figures. The list on page 33 gives some idea of the amount of 'hidden' sugar in typical foods.

The world production of sugar has grown from 1½ million tons in 1850 to the present level of 75 million tons per annum. In the U.K. we now eat 25 times the amount of sugar we ate 200 years ago. The Englishman of 1780 would have taken two years to eat the same amount of sugar his 1980 counterpart eats in one month.

The intake of sugar is not spread evenly over the population, as it has been shown that there is a disproportionately high consumption in young people, the highest consumption being in twelve to fourteen year olds. Children in general eat twice as much sugar and starch as the national average, and consumption in the U.K. is currently the highest in the world. This depressing picture indicates that the average child in this country obtains between 25 and 35 per cent of his/her total calories from sugar.

Figure 2. Sugar consumption in Britain.

Table 3. Sugar Content of Food

Food	Amount	Sugar Equivalent in teaspoonsful
Chocolate fudge	4 oz (100g)	14
Chewing gum	1 stick	3
Chocolate cake	1 medium slice	14
Sponge cake	1 medium slice	6
Doughnut	Small	4
Average biscuit	1 biscuit	2
Baked Custard	½ cupful	4
Ice cream	5 oz (150g)	6
Apple pie	1 medium slice	12
Chocolate sauce	1 teaspoonful	4½
Jam	1 tablespoonful	3
Honey	1 tablespoonful	3
Cocoa (all milk)	1 cupful	5
Coca-Cola	1 bottle	4

Why All the Fuss?

Professor John Yudkin in his book *Pure, White and Deadly* makes two very significant statements which are worth quoting. First, '. . . there is no physiological requirement for sugar', and second, '. . . if only a small fraction of what is already known about the facts of sugar were to be revealed in relation to any other material used as a food additive, the material would promptly be banned'.[9]

How has the confusion over sugar arisen? To most people it is a necessary source of energy and we are told 'it helps us work, rest and play'. Glucose drinks are given to aid convalescence, barley sugar and chocolate are prescribed for fatigue and glucose tablets recommended for sportsmen. The confusion arises perhaps from the use of the word 'sugar' for, as I have already shown, there are many sugars. Sugar as glucose *is* needed as an essential fuel for the body, especially the nervous system, but we do not need to *eat* glucose. The glucose should enter our bodies as an integral part of various unrefined and complex foods, gradually being broken down in a step by step process before passing into the blood as glucose. It may also be made available, if required, by the conversion of glycogen stored in the liver. In this way, the available glucose is utilized for energy as required, or stored if not required. Eating large amounts of glucose (as sugar, etc.) bypasses the normal digestive step ladder and presents the body with a substance it simply cannot use. In a natural environment, we can obtain sugar only by eating unrefined cereals or fruit, and our normal appetite would not allow us to eat more than a limited amount. This would be digested and the glucose gradually released.

The refining of starch has led to a situation where we can eat large amounts of concentrated sugar. Unfortunately, the human digestive system has yet to adapt to the changes in our dietary habits. As a result, the modern diet is very different from the ideal diet for man that has evolved over several million years.

One important factor that allows for the high consumption of sugar, is its cheapness. In the sixteenth century the cost of sugar was equivalent to the present cost of caviar, and, in fact, its price has fallen to only 0.5 per cent of the fifteenth century price. In spite of this, the income from the sale of sugar and confectionery in the U.K. is at present around £2,000 million per year.

Dead Calories
Sugar is either eaten in addition to a normal diet or it replaces the more valuable foods in the diet. Approximately 500 calories a day are supplied by sugar in the typical British diet. It follows that sugar eaters will either (a) put on weight, or (b) be deprived of food that is replaced by sugar.

It is not the brief of this book to detail the harmful effects of sugar but, as hypoglycaemic patients have a craving for sugar, they are usually prone to the effects of a high sugar diet. The damaging effects of sugar are well reviewed in many publications.[9][20][48]

5
MIGRAINE

Symptoms
Someone once wrote, 'There are headaches and there are migraine headaches'. It is perhaps wrong to classify migraine as a headache, although the word 'migraine' implies hemi-cranial or half-head. It should be stated, before going further, that a headache is never the only symptom experienced during a migraine attack. The complete syndrome, sometimes termed 'common migraine', involves various components grouped as follows.

Headache
Usually one-sided but may be both sides of the head. Great variations exist in severity and duration, but rarely less than two to three hours and can last seven to ten days. (I have encountered patients who have awakened with a headache every morning.) Intensity can vary enormously from a constant dull ache to an incapacitating, throbbing and violent pain. Pain may be above the eyes, at the base of the skull and may occasionally travel to the face and jaw, producing symptoms similar to trigeminal neuralgia.

Nausea
Migraine is often referred to as a sick headache, for nausea invariably accompanies the headache. There may be a tendency to vomit or a feeling of nausea associated with the smell or even the sight of food. Other symptoms frequently accompany the nausea, including heartburn, over-salivation, hiccup, belching and retching. Sometimes the vomiting signals the end of the migraine. If, however, vomiting is severe, protracted and accompanied by heavy sweating, the resulting fluid depletion may lead to prostration.

Appearance
In severe cases the patient has the look of someone in shock, with pale drawn features. There may be puffiness and oedema of the face, often around one eye or to the side of the mouth. At the onset of a migraine the face may be bright red, suddenly turning pale.

Visual Symptoms
A variety of symptoms affect the eyes, the commonest being photophobia (sensitivity to light), blurring of vision or blood-shot eyes.

Digestive Symptoms
Some migraine sufferers experience cramp-like pains in the stomach, constipation, distension with occasional diarrhoea and sharp colic-type pain as the attack progresses. This effect is sometimes termed 'abdominal migraine'.

Sinus Symptoms
Symptoms similar to hay fever or chronic rhinitis may precede a migraine attack. Nasal stuffiness and loss of smell may be experienced with frequent sneezing.

Fatigue
A frequent symptom of migraine is a feeling of lethargy and drowsiness with occasional pronounced muscular weakness and heaviness. Insomnia is common, the brief periods of sleep being very deep and dream-filled.

Balance
For a variety of reasons migraine sufferers often feel dizzy or faint and may have difficulty in focusing their eyes.

Water Retention
A characteristic of the migraine patient is the tendency to retain fluid during an attack. The mechanism of this will be discussed in a later chapter and is due to an imbalance in the sodium/potassium ratio.

Emotional Changes
Not surprisingly, the moods of the person experiencing a migraine attack will vary with the symptoms. There are,

however, predictable mood changes that are symptomatic of migraine. These include: initial anxiety followed by depression; severe agitation and fits of bad temper, followed by despair and apathy if the attack is protracted.

Other Symptoms

The severity of a migraine attack can lead to some very unusual symptoms, including: nose bleeds; hot flushings; extreme sensitivity to noise; and a distortion of certain tastes and smells.

Many migraine attacks are preceded by what is termed an 'aura' or classical migraine. In early medical literature this strange effect was likened to visions or trances and has been recognized as an early warning of migraine for over two thousand years. The aura may be experienced as a mild hallucination or a dream-like loss of contact with reality. To most sufferers, however, it is simply an awareness that an attack is imminent, yet most migraine patients find it very difficult to explain the exact nature of their 'warning'.

Many different types of migraine have been defined according to their pattern of cause and frequency. It has often been stated that there is no such thing as a typical migraine and those who have never experienced a migraine attack or do not have a migraine sufferer in their immediate family, are sometimes puzzled and unsympathetic about the fuss caused by 'just a headache'. The nearest experience to a migraine attack for many of us is a severe hangover. All the components are there – the sensitive eyes, feeling of sickness, a splitting headache and a tendency to jump at slight noises. These symptoms are usually accompanied by a feeling of mental and physical lethargy and a feeling that it would be preferable if one were allowed to quietly die. On a more serious note, the migraine sufferer and the drunkard are both suffering from an imbalance in their metabolism. For different reasons their blood glucose level has fallen and precipitated the distressing symptoms they are experiencing. Small wonder that the majority of migraine sufferers cannot tolerate alcohol.

The actual cause of a migraine headache at the site (within the brain) is thought to be a localized vaso-dilation (increased pressure within the blood vessels causing them to swell). This results in pressure, irritation and pain and, as the cranial nerves become affected, problems are referred to the eyes, ears, liver and stomach. To understand the link between this vaso-dilation and low blood sugar, it is necessary to discuss, step by step, how one affects the other.

Migraine and Blood Sugar

Glucose is almost the only fuel required by nerve tissue and, understandably, the body always gives priority to the supply of fuel to the brain and nervous system. To facilitate this, automatic compensatory reactions take place when the glucose level drops, for, under normal conditions, the total glucose concentration within the brain would be exhausted within 10-15 minutes if glucose were not readily available. (It has been shown that a drop of as little as five per cent in the glucose requirement to the brain creates symptoms of nerve deprivation, i.e. neuroglycopenia). The glucose supplied to the brain is topped up by an automatic increase in blood volume. In other words, reduced quality leads to increased quantity. In this way, although the concentration of glucose has been reduced, sufficient glucose is made available to brain and nerve tissue by the simple expedient of increasing the flow of blood to the brain. Unfortunately, if this compensatory mechanism operates too frequently on a regular basis, owing to the repeated lowering of the blood glucose level, the nerve tissues become oversensitive from the pressure of the bulging blood vessels passing through them. It is this increased blood pressure that creates the headache and other symptoms.

In a group of 35 migraine sufferers given a six-hour glucose tolerance test, all 35 were diagnosed as hypoglycaemic.[10] In my practice I have found that, of the migraine patients tested for low blood sugar, 92 per cent were confirmed as hypoglycaemic. It would seem that, although migraine is a complex and distressing problem with many trigger factors, the principal underlying cause is an imbalance in the blood glucose level.

Migraine attacks frequently follow a predictable pattern. They may occur just before or during menstruation, after eating chocolate, cheese or drinking alcohol. A common trigger is fatigue or stress, and even strenuous exercise can initiate an attack. Many sufferers from migraine and lesser headaches find that the commonest pattern is the headache on wakening. Often the headache will occur at almost exactly the same time each morning. This is not difficult to understand when one realizes that the level of blood sugar drops to its lowest point in the early hours between 3 a.m. and 5 a.m. By the same token, the asthma sufferer becomes wheezy and distressed early in the morning, for the same causative factors prevail.

A tendency exists in medical circles to attribute the cause of migraine to a great variety of factors, varying from food allergy and sensitivity to stress and personality problems. There are obviously many different causes of headaches, some trivial, others extremely serious. There seems little doubt, however, that the type of headache known as migraine is, in the vast majority of cases, due to blood sugar imbalance.

6

ASTHMA AND HAY FEVER

Asthma was first described 1,800 years ago by Aretaeus the Cappadocian, significantly the same physician who identified the symptoms of diabetes.

Causes of Asthma

Although these two conditions frequently existed in the same family, it was always assumed that a genetic imbalance in some way became split, producing either diabetes or asthma. In spite of the common occurrence of both conditions in the same family, they never occurred together in one person (except in very rare cases which will be discussed later). The common denominator in the asthma patient and the diabetic patient is blood sugar imbalance, the asthmatic having hypoglycaemia and the diabetic having hyperglycaemia. It should be said, however, that not all hypoglycaemics have asthma, nor do all asthmatics have hypoglycaemia. There is a type of asthma known as psychic or 'stress' asthma that has a psychological cause. However, the evidence to support the view that hypolgycaemia is the main cause of asthma is overwhelming. (Between the years 1959 and 1966 the death rate from asthma increased *eight times* among the 10-14 year olds – just the age for highest sugar consumption.)[11]

The medical view that asthma is triggered by an allergen, e.g. pollen or a stress situation, is not supported by the timing of a typical asthma attack. Most asthmatics experience symptoms in the early hours, often being awakened by the distressing symptoms of suffocation and breathlessness. Significantly, the pollen count drops to its lowest level at night and the sufferer cannot be under a great deal of stress when he or she is asleep in bed! The blood sugar level, however, is at its lowest level between 3 a.m. and 5 a.m., hence the onset of symptoms at this time.

If we accept the notion that asthmatics suffer from low blood sugar – where is the evidence? Diabetics are thought to be protected from asthma by their high blood sugar level, for the only condition leading to a person having both asthma and diabetes is that of dysinsulinism. Here the alteration of high and low blood sugar leads to symptoms of both disorders. This extremely rare condition is thought to be due to a delay in insulin production (leading to high blood sugar) followed by an inappropriate excess of insulin (low blood sugar). This imbalance can be identified and diagnosed by the use of a six-hour glucose tolerance test.

It is interesting to note that the drugs commonly used for asthma relief act by raising the blood sugar, e.g. cortisone, adrenalin, etc. Furthermore, the habit of prescribing sugar or glucose injections to stop an asthma attack only serves to alleviate the symptoms for a short time. The resulting rise in blood sugar level is rapidly followed by a drop in the sugar level due to stimulation of the pancreas and the insulin reaction, and the asthma symptoms reappear.

In 1939, Joslyn, a renowned authority on diabetes, drew attention to the 'protective role' of diabetes in relation to asthma. He noted that many asthmatics who develop diabetes rapidly lose their asthma symptoms.[12]

Many glands in the body produce substances that have an antagonistic or opposite effect to insulin. One of these is the thyroid which produces a hormone called thyroxine. As long ago as 1913, asthma was frequently treated by prescribing thyroid extract, as it was found that many asthmatics had underactive thyroids. This reduced secretion of thyroxine led to an oversecretion of insulin which, in turn, resulted in hypoglycaemia. Conversely, it was observed that patients with overactive or toxic thyroids often lost their asthma symptoms, and removal of the enlarged gland caused a return of the asthma.

The mechanism whereby a decrease in the blood sugar level triggers off the symptoms of asthma (and indeed many other allergies) is not fully understood. The results of recent research work, however, suggest that the substance histamine, which affects cell permeability and tissue fluid balance, is present in abnormal amounts in the blood of allergic persons.

Significantly, the stressful, hypoglycaemic patient also has an elevated blood histamine level, possibly due to the over-production of histamine by the body when under stress. Although this is an extremely complex process, it is thought that the breakdown and utilization of protein from body tissue, accelerated under conditions of stress, leads to the release of excess histamine into the blood.

Under normal conditions, the body, in its wisdom, has a safeguard to avoid excessive build-up of histamine. It releases a substance from the liver known as histaminase which destroys the surplus histamine. If, however, the liver is congested or damaged owing to wrong diet, drug abuse, alcoholism or hepatitis, then this safeguard is weakened or removed and the histamine remains high. (The relationship between liver congestion and the characteristic high starch diet of the hypoglycaemic is well known. The excessive consumption of starch leads to a surplus of glucose which the body converts to glycogen for storage in the liver and other tissues. If, however, the intake of starch is out of proportion to the utilization of glycogen, there is an inevitable build-up in the liver leading to congestion and malfunction.) On the face of it, the taking of antihistamine drugs would seem to be a simple solution to this problem. Many investigators have shown, however, that the use of drugs to reduce the histamine level is not the answer, as the drugs themselves can cause further liver damage because of their toxicity.[13]

Hay Fever
Although the symptoms of hay fever are not as serious as asthma, it is nonetheless a distressing condition. Research has shown that the hay fever sufferer also shows a characteristic blood sugar imbalance. As the area affected in hay fever involves the nose, eyes and upper respiratory system, it is inevitable that hay fever is usually triggered off by airborne irritation, e.g. pollen, household dust, etc. Although not so easily affected by food or stress as in asthma, the role of various trigger factors in hay fever can be more significant than in asthma.

In my experience there is a background, low profile hypoglycaemia in most hay fever sufferers, which is expressed in a seasonal sensitivity to dust or pollen. The medically defined condition known as chronic rhinitis or sinusitis can be seen as chronic hay fever. The sufferer experiences stuffed nose and inflamed eyes, particularly in the morning on waking. He cannot tolerate dust of any kind, the irritation from which sets up a whole series of sneezes.

There is a need, therefore, in all the respiratory/allergy problems, to consider the possibility of low blood sugar as the prime cause, irrespective of the types of trigger factors or the diversity of symptoms.

We cannot escape the fact that correct nutrition should be the first consideration in successfully treating these distressing complaints.

7

RHEUMATISM AND ARTHRITIS

Rheumatism and arthritis are broad terms to describe a whole family of muscle and joint problems. Arthritis means simply 'inflammation of the joints'. The commonest members of this large family are osteo-arthritis, gout and rheumatoid-arthritis.

Osteo-arthritis can be seen as accelerated wear and tear and, not surprisingly, affects chiefly the weight-bearing joints, e.g. knees and hips, and the joints involved in the most activity, e.g. thumb and wrist.

Gout is essentially an expression of a biochemical imbalance involving a gradual silting up of certain joints by crystals of uric acid. This occurs as a result of an imbalance in the blood leading to a precipitation of excessive uric acid into crystals causing swelling, redness and severe pain. The joints mainly affected are the weight-bearing joints of the lower extremities, especially the great toes and the knees. Although the excessive eating of certain proteins and wines is an important factor in gout, (being almost an epidemic amongst the wealthy classes in the seventeenth and eighteenth centuries, so much so that special gout stools were available upon which the Regency gentlemen could rest their painful swollen feet), there are, however, other causes of gout apart from nutritional imbalances.

Rheumatoid arthritis is the most widespread and perhaps the least understood of the arthritis family. The characteristic symptoms include fatigue; pain; distortion and swelling of the extremity joints – especially the hands; loss of power in muscles and eventual disablement in many cases. Several theories have been offered to explain the causes of rheumatoid arthritis, ranging from inherited tendencies to stress and the inevitable virus. Current medical thinking, however, suggests that the condition represents a breakdown in the body's antibody system, leading to a situation where the sufferer develops antibodies to his own tissues. Instead of the antibodies fighting bacteria or virus they act against the body. This is known as an auto-immune disease.

Treatment

A recent popular publication on arthritis and rheumatism lists the treatment for arthritis as follows:[14]

1. Rest.
2. Occupational therapy and appliances; adaptations to the home.
3. Splints and plasters.
4. Physiotherapy.
5. Drugs.
6. Surgery.

It is interesting to note that no mention is made of correct nutrition.

Osteo-arthritis is treated mainly with heat, exercise, physiotherapy, drugs and injections and, as a last resort, surgical joint replacement. Very little attention is paid to joint misalignment, tissue health, diet and weight control.

Traditionally, gout was treated by avoidance of the proteins that lead to the uric acid build-up. These include certain fish, liver, sweetbreads, brain and red wine. This 'low purine' diet unfortunately only controls and does very little to cure. Modern drug treatment is equally superficial, drugs being prescribed to reduce the formation of uric acid (e.g. allopurinol) and to increase loss of uric acid via the kidneys. For the greater majority of patients suffering from the various joint problems discussed, the treatment is usually analgesics or anti-inflammatory drugs. For many it is a waiting game as the masked symptoms gradually worsen to the point of incapacity or surgery.

Perhaps the most controversial treatment is the use of steroids (cortisone, prednisolone and ACTH) as they are considered by many to be miracle drugs, and by others to be very harmful. It may be worth looking more closely at this particular treatment.

Cortisone

Cortisone, and hydro-cortisone, are natural substances produced by the cortex of the adrenal glands. Their main role, as explained in Chapter 8, is in carbohydrate metabolism. Since their original discovery as a possible treatment for arthritis in the 1940s, a bewildering range of synthetic materials with similar structure has been produced. Perhaps the best known is prednisone and prednisolone.

ACTH (Corticotropin)

This substance is not produced by the adrenal glands and is, in fact, released by the anterior pituitary gland in the forehead. This master gland releases various substances that activate or stimulate other glands. (One author described the pituitary gland as 'the conductor of the glandular orchestra'.) The action of ACTH is to stimulate the adrenal cortex. In this roundabout way, cortisone production is also increased. ACTH is considered less harmful than cortisone, for it creates fewer side-effects.

Effects and Side-Effects

As long ago as 1936, the Canadian physiologist Professor Hans Selye noted that large amounts of corticosteroid hormones were produced as part of the body's adaptation to stress.[15] With prolonged stress, there can occur adrenal exhaustion with the inevitable reduction in cortisone flow. It is not fully understood how cortisone affects joints, but we do know it has an important role in protecting joints against inflammation. Hence the dramatic improvement in arthritic patients when they take cortisone. Significantly, most arthritic sufferers have a history of stress which would, of course, deplete their own cortisone level. When cortisone was first used for arthritis, doctors were reassured that if the body produced sufficient cortisone, simply providing additional cortisone would not bring about improvement. Therefore, when cortisone was prescribed for arthritic patients and produced apparently miraculous changes, it was assumed that arthritic patients were deficient in adrenal hormones.

Unfortunately, time has shown that the body does not need extra cortisone, and side-effects – many quite devastating – are caused by regularly taking cortisone and other steroids. A safer and more logical approach is to provide adequate nutrition to meet the demands of stress and, in addition, take substances that we know increase the body's own cortisone flow. Dr Roger Williams, the discoverer of the B vitamin pantothenic acid, advocates this important vitamin as a treatment for arthritis and gout since, without it, cortisone cannot be produced.[16] Research work has shown that the adrenal glands actually shrivel and the hormone flow is markedly reduced when pantothenic acid is not available.

Arthritis and Low Blood Sugar

You may well comment at this stage 'Very interesting, but what has this to do with low blood sugar?'

In 1906, Francis Hare, a British psychiatrist, published a massive book on food ecology called *The Food Factor in Disease*. In this he stated that many conditions, including migraine, asthma, eczema, epilepsy, angina, gout and rheumatoid arthritis were caused by the excessive consumption of starch and sugar. This view was based on his observations that patients on such a diet showed dramatic symptom improvement when they reduced their starch and replaced the sugary foods with protein. He also found that patients on high sugar diets were, in fact, addicted to sugar, and severe withdrawal symptoms were noted after reducing their sugar intake for a few days. This malaise and depression would often cause the patient to return to his sugar after which he would feel better.

Medical workers have never been quick to adopt new ideas, and the concept that diet in any way influenced the cause of disease was quite revolutionary. Unfortunately, this notion still pervades present medical attitudes. Although, perhaps, his terminology was slightly different, Dr Hare was anticipating Seale Harris's theories by thirty years. He was, of course, describing exactly the cause, symptoms and withdrawal effects of the typical hypoglycaemic sufferer.

Hormones

It is an interesting fact that many of the conditions attributed to low blood sugar improve during pregnancy. This particularly applies to migraine, epilepsy, gastric ulcers and rheumatoid arthritis. Dr Abrahamson, an American authority on hypo-glycaemia, attributes this to '. . . the large amounts of pituitary hormones and cortisone which, being antagonistic to insulin, will tend to allow the glucose level to increase, and conditions in which low blood sugar are found will therefore tend to become milder.[17] I have noticed in my practice that arthritic patients tend to follow the characteristic pattern of low blood sugar sufferers, often improving dramatically during pregnancy but, conversely, experiencing a severe flare-up of symptoms immediately before periods. Although very little work has been carried out to show a link between pre-menstrual tension, arthritis symptoms and low blood sugar, there is an interesting clue to a possible common factor.

Calcium

It has been known for over thirty years that low blood sugar is accompanied by a low calcium level in the blood. A characteristic of low blood sugar is, as we know, a tendency to hyperinsulinism with resulting overactivity in the stomach secretions. Unless the gastric acid (pH) is normal, calcium is not absorbed. This can create a situation where rheumatic patients with low blood

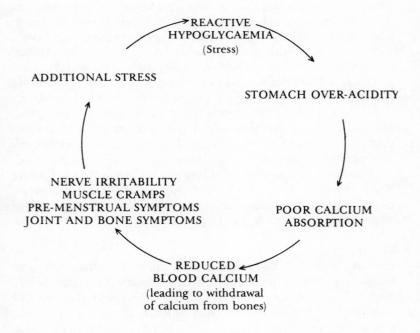

Figure 3. The role of calcium in reactive hypoglycaemia.

sugar may be withdrawing calcium from the bones to maintain a normal level of blood calcium. Another aspect of the role of calcium in hypoglycaemia is that a reduced blood calcium level leads to a hyper-sensitivity and irritability of the nervous system. This can cause muscle cramps and spasm.

Although the body contains more calcium than any other mineral, the absorption of calcium is very inefficient for only 10-30 per cent of the calcium consumed is absorbed. With this in mind, it is worth noting that, under stress, absorption is decreased and excretion increased. (The role of calcium and low blood sugar is expressed in diagram form in Figure 3.)

To summarize, the low level of calcium in the blood of arthritic patients may well be attributed to the low blood sugar and the high insulin found in their blood. The vicious circle is complete, for a calcium deficiency can lead to weak bones, muscle cramps and nerve irritability. This irritability can lead to further stress and resulting hypoglycaemia.

Pre-menstrual Tension
Women patients with rheumatoid arthritis invariably feel an aggravation of symptoms prior to and during periods. The calcium level drops steadily and predictably eight or ten days before the period, causing pre-menstrual tension, depression and headache. Dr Roger Williams has listed the symptoms of calcium deficiency as anxiety neurosis, fatigue, insomnia and tension.[16] The system reacts to this situation as it would to stress, producing extra cortisone and, inevitably, fluid retention. The muscle cramps associated with calcium deficiency may affect the emptying womb, causing abdominal pain and spasm.

You will begin to understand why calcium is so often prescribed for low blood sugar, and why rheumatoid arthritis should, in many cases, be seen as yet another condition related to hypoglycaemia.

Osteo-arthritis and Gout
The role of calcium in relation to low blood sugar and rheumatoid arthritis, as described above, also applies to many of the other conditions in the arthritis family. In osteo-arthritis, the weakened bones and muscle stiffness due, in part, to calcium imbalance, play a considerable role in the joint wear and tear. Additional factors in low blood sugar

patients are circulatory impairment, fatigue and frequent overweight, all of which contribute to the osteo-arthritis symptoms.

Gout is closely related to arthritis and, contrary to medical thinking, it is not simply caused by an excessive amount of uric acid in the blood. Dr Williams points out, 'The mere presence of high uric acid in the blood is not enough to cause gout, its salts must be precipitated in and around the joints and this does not always happen in individuals who have a high content of uric acid in the blood'.[16] This was confirmed by his finding that only one patient in ten with a high blood uric acid level showed symptoms of gout. He further showed that pantothenic acid can convert the excess uric acid into harmless, easily-excreted substances, and suggested that the individual's dietary requirements could provide the clue to this puzzling condition. Although little work has been done relating gout to low blood sugar, Joslin – the authority on diabetes – has observed that gout is very rare in diabetics.[12] Furthermore, treatment with cortisone (a substance that we know will increase the blood sugar concentration) invariably improves the symptoms of gout.

It would be a mistake for me to suggest that arthritic conditions are entirely due to low blood sugar. Many other factors are involved, including inheritance, anaemia, vitamin C levels, fats in the blood, endocrine imbalance and individual metabolic requirements. There is, however, considerable evidence available to suggest that many arthritic sufferers have associated low blood sugar, and that the treatment of the blood sugar imbalance frequently alleviates the arthritic symptoms.

8

DIABETES AND HYPOGLYCAEMIA

When discussing low blood sugar with patients in an attempt to explain its cause and treatment, I find a useful starting point is to ask the question, 'Are you familiar with diabetes?' The usual answer is 'Yes, although not in detail'. Even a rough understanding of diabetes aids the understanding of hypoglycaemia for, although the two conditions are opposite, the problems involved are also, in a way, complementary.

The symptoms of diabetes were noted almost 3,500 years ago, whilst hypoglycaemia was first recorded and defined a mere fifty years ago. As I have said, hypoglycaemia due to simple hyperinsulinism can be seen as an exact medical opposite to diabetes, a mirror image, as one is high blood sugar (diabetes) and the other low blood sugar (hypoglycaemia).

In order to understand how hypoglycaemia can develop into diabetes in later life, how the two conditions can exist together and why the diets prescribed for the two problems are remarkably similar, it may help to take a closer look at diabetes.

Diabetes: Its Early Study and Treatment
The excessive passing of urine, an obvious sign of diabetes, was the subject of an Egyptian papyrus written around 3,500 years ago called the Papyrus Ebeas. It gives detailed prescriptions for medicines to reduce the urine output. Close to A.D. 200 Aretaeus the Cappadocian produced the first precise description of diabetes. He also described tetanus, chest and heart problems and epilepsy. The word 'diabaiton' derives from the Greek word meaning 'to stand with legs apart like a ladder'. Aretaeus used this word for the symptoms of diabetes as he considered that 'the fluid uses the patient's body as a ladder to

escape downwards'. The modern word 'diabetes' evolved from this original Greek word.

In the fifteenth century the word 'mellitus' (meaning honey) was added to diabetes. The Latin word for honey (mel), being the basis for mellitus, was used to describe the sweet-tasting urine of the diabetic. In spite of the earlier observations, it was not until the end of the nineteenth century that some understanding of the cause of the strange symptoms of diabetes was achieved. A Russian named Oscar Minkowski showed that the removal of a dog's pancreas caused the dog to die from symptoms exactly similar to those of the diabetic sufferer.

With the field of study narrowed down to the pancreas, it was not long before workers were able to isolate the insulin secreted from small glands on the pancreas (later named the Islets of Langerhans) as the key to diabetes. In 1869 the glands were identified in diabetic patients. The ensuing race to discover and isolate insulin was won by a young Canadian doctor named Banting who, with his colleague Charles Best, showed that pancreatic extract (insulin) could be used to prolong the life of diabetic dogs. The next small step involved the relatively simple process of purifying insulin for general use.

When considering diabetes one may ask, 'If the body cannot deal with sugar owing to a poor insulin response, why not simply reduce or avoid sugar and allow the pancreas to rest?' Unfortunately we cannot avoid absorbing sugar for, although carbohydrates (starches) are completely converted to glucose, fats and proteins are also partially converted as follows. [17]

Table 4: Conversion of Food Groups to Glucose

Food	Percentage Converted
Carbohydrates	100
Fats	10
Proteins	50

It would therefore be necessary to avoid all foods if we were to prevent glucose entering the bloodstream.

When the earlier doctors treated their diabetic patients

they were obliged (in the absence of insulin therapy) to adjust their patients' diet as best they could. The protein requirements are predictable and fixed and could not be safely varied as proteins are used for tissue repair, antibody production and many other vital processes. It follows that the only adjustment that could be safely achieved was by reducing carbohydrates and increasing fats. The complete and safe breakdown of fats requires a minimal amount of carbohydrate and, in the type of diet prescribed to the diabetic of the pre-insulin period, there occurred an inevitable build-up of fat residues, in particular acetone and diacetic acid. This excess of acetone in the blood causes a reduction in the blood alkaline reserve and eventual coma. At the same time, acetone spills over into the urine where it can be detected. This condition is known as 'acidosis'. The acetone is also expelled via the lungs giving a characteristic smell to the breath. Before insulin was available, a diabetic patient inevitably died of acidosis, in spite of special diets and careful nursing.

Fat Absorption
An additional problem for the diabetic, and still a problem even with modern treatment, is that of fat absorption. Without insulin the liver cannot store excess sugar, which it normally does by converting the sugar to glycogen. After the liver is saturated with converted sugar (as glycogen), the excess glycogen is converted into fat and stored, usually in muscle tissue. The liver is enlarged with the deposits of stored glycogen (owing to excess consumption *or* insufficient insulin availability). Once the 'storage' areas (i.e. liver and muscle) are saturated, the excess fat overspills into the bloodstream. It is the build-up of various fats in the blood of the diabetic that leads to the two main secondary effects in mature diabetics. These are diabetic retinitis (retinopathy) and diabetic gangrene. Both these unpleasant conditions are in part due to a narrowing and thickening of small blood vessels. Not surprisingly, many diabetics are also obese owing to the store of spare fat in various tissues. High blood pressure, strokes and heart attacks are more frequent than among non-diabetics. Other complications include athero-sclerosis, fatty livers and cataracts.

The tailoring of the insulin dosage to carbohydrate intake

Figure 4. An outline of carbohydrate absorption.

can unfortunately lead to a situation where diabetic patients need to eat more starch to balance the insulin in order to avoid 'hypo-ing' (hypoglycaemia due to excess insulin). This situation can lead to a further reduction in pancreatic efficiency, and a vicious circle is set up.

Blood Sugar Levels

The normal blood sugar fasting level is about 70-100mg per 100cc of blood. However, as we are not normally fasting for periods of longer than two to three hours, it must be seen that the normal level of blood sugar during an active day would be considerably higher, i.e. 120-140mg. As the available glucose reserve in the blood is only equivalent to two teaspoonsful of sugar, it is essential for the body to be able to draw off some reserves of sugar as well as control excess sugar. The food is broken down and passed to the liver; in a similar way the insulin, when released, is also passed to the liver. This enables the small amount of insulin that remains after the excess glucose is converted to glycogen to pass throughout the body assisting the utilization of blood glucose.

We should know the events that follow the eating of carbohydrates, for then we may more easily understand high and low blood sugar conditions (see Figure 4).

If a situation arises where the blood glucose concentration exceeds 165 mg per 100 cc, the excess spills over into the urine. This overflow level is known as the renal (kidneys') threshold, and can be seen as a normal compensatory device to rid the blood of surplus glucose. The kidneys' 'threshold' may, however, be reduced to the point where sugar appears in the urine despite *normal* levels being present in the blood. This is known as renal diabetes and is not an expression of sugar-insulin imbalance.

At the other extreme, damaged or diseased kidneys may be unable to pass any sugar into the urine, leading to a high blood sugar level being completely masked. A true assessment of high or low blood sugar is, therefore, only obtained by measuring the blood sugar level. The most informative and valuable test is the six-hour glucose tolerance test (discussed in Chapter 10).

Adrenal Glands

There is one further piece in the jigsaw that illustrates blood sugar levels, this being the role of the adrenal glands. These glands are located near the kidneys and produce several important hormones. The centre of the gland, the medulla, secretes adrenalin (epinephrine). The outer layer, the cortex, produces cortisol (hydrocortisone), cortisone and several other less important substances. Under normal conditions, the available glucose is utilized by the body for energy and the blood glucose level drops. This lowering of blood glucose stimulates the secretions of the adrenal cortex, and the hormones released have an opposite effect to insulin. They are passed in the blood to the liver, where they facilitate the conversion of the stored glycogen into glucose. It can be seen that this balances the action of insulin and, in normal health, an optimum blood sugar level is maintained. The adrenalin secreted by the centre of the adrenal gland has a similar effect. The rate of use is, however, very different, for adrenalin can be seen as part of a 'back-up' or emergency system. It is secreted by the gland when the body requires a rapid glucose increase to provide an energy surge. The pulse then quickens and the blood pressure rises, allowing the increased glucose to reach the muscles rapidly. In animals, this provides available energy literally for fight or flight. Unfortunately, in 'civilized' human beings, the mechanism is triggered far too frequently owing to physical or mental stress, and the subsequent adrenal exhaustion can cause a variety of problems, in particular the lowered output of cortisone, related closely to the onset of joint problems, particularly rheumatoid arthritis.

To a lesser extent, the stored glycogen in the muscles is also affected by insulin and adrenal hormone levels, but the greater activity occurs in the liver.

9

LOW BLOOD SUGAR: THE 20TH CENTURY EPIDEMIC

'Epidemic' is defined in the *Oxford Dictionary* as 'prevalent among community at special time'. The symptoms and illness caused by low blood sugar are certainly prevalent among the community, the special time being the twentieth century. Considerable debate surrounds the question of whether hypoglycaemia is a common condition expressed in a multitude of disorders, or a very rare condition that is falsely blamed for the disorders. The answer to this question surely lies in the frequency of diagnosis of hypoglycaemia. Doctors who regularly use glucose tolerance tests as a diagnostic tool have offered figures ranging from 10-50 per cent of the population for the incidence of hypoglycaemia. Data from a 1966-67 survey carried out by the U.S. Department of Health, Education and Welfare showed that 66,000 persons from a total of 134,000 were hypoglycaemic.[18] When Dr C R Harper tested 175 United Airlines pilots, 44 showed evidence of hypoglycaemia.[19] Dr Atkins, the American authority on nutrition and disease, who has tested many thousands of patients with the six-hour glucose tolerance test, has found that one in ten patients has been diagnosed as hypoglycaemic.[20] More will be said about the glucose tolerance test and the diagnosis of hypoglycaemia in later chapters. Sufficient to say, however, that this condition is certainly not rare.

This chapter deals with the many less obvious conditions that can be caused by hypoglycaemia. Most of them are on the increase in 'civilized' countries.

Sugar Consumption
The great diseases of the previous centuries, e.g. T.B., cholera, syphilis, diphtheria and typhoid have been virtually eliminated,

but this century has seen an increase in the degenerative and mental disorders. Diabetes, asthma, rheumatoid arthritis, heart conditions, cancer and obesity are all increasing and can be seen as the characteristic diseases of this century. It is significant that the increased incidence of these conditions correlates with the increased sugar consumption in this century.

Although it should be stated that other factors may also cause these disorders, there is much evidence to show that declining health affects a country or community when sugar consumption increases. Dr T L Cleave has described conditions caused by taking excess sugar as the 'saccharine disease'.[21] He has shown that the introduction of sugar to primitive societies in various parts of the world has resulted in a rapid increase in diabetes (which so often follows hypoglycaemia), stomach ulcers and coronary heart disease. He has observed that the increased consumption of sugar in Western nations causes a corresponding increase in mortality from diabetes. (In the Metropolitan Life Insurance Company's causes of death statistics, diabetes in 1900 was twenty-seventh on the list. By 1950 it was the third most common cause of death.) Dr Cleave states that, '. . . the key to the causation of coronary thrombosis lies in the causation of diabetes'.

The Heart and Hypoglycaemia

Coronary heart disease is now the number-one killer. How can it be that a condition which a mere century ago was attributed to old age and therefore rarely mentioned in medical text books is now responsible for the death of tens of thousands of apparently healthy men and women, many of whom were in their late twenties and thirties? The answer lies in the massive increase in the consumption of sugar and the imbalance in sugar and fat metabolism that results from this consumption. A lot of research has been carried out to show that hypoglycaemia and a high sugar diet contribute to various heart disorders. In 1933 Dr Paton wrote in *The Lancet* that the rise in sugar consumption may be the cause of heart disease and heart attacks. He pointed out that the 'clinically associated' conditions of obesity, arterio-sclerosis and diabetes are also on the increase. Dr R. A. Ahrens of the University of Maryland showed conclusively in a number of animal studies that increased sugar consumption shortened the average life-span.[22]

He added weight to the cholesterol myth by concluding that the huge worldwide increase in heart disease increases in rough proportion to the increase in sugar consumption, and not fat consumption.

The heart specialists, White and Stare, wrote in 1954, 'No disease has come so quickly from obscurity to the place coronary heart disease now occupies'. (i.e. Heart disease is the primary cause of death in the U.S.A.) Many workers have shown the correlation between hypoglycaemia and the incidence of heart disease, including Dr B. Sandler. His paper in the *Homeostasis* (Autumn, 1974)[23] showed that angina and coronary heart disease are frequently caused by a sharp fall in the blood sugar level.

Cholesterol

Surely a word to strike terror in most people. For years it has been blamed as the single main cause of heart disease. As a result, patients have been encouraged to reduce the fat in their diet to dangerously low levels, and to avoid valuable protein foods. Yet to date, no evidence is available to show that eating cholesterol actually affects our blood cholesterol levels. Indeed, many patients with an inherited high cholesterol level have perfectly sound hearts, and many coronary victims have normal cholesterol levels.

It has long been assumed that most overweight people have an imbalance in their carbohydrate metabolism. Insulin is sometimes called the fattening hormone simply because it promotes the storage of starch and fat. (The stored starch is known as glycogen and the stored fat is termed triglycerides.) Insulin also converts fatty acids back to stored fat. Not surprisingly, those of us with hypoglycaemia and hyper-insulinism tend to be overweight. So the patient with low blood sugar craves sugar, the high sugar diet produces insulin which causes fat to be stored and eventually spill over into the blood. Finally the excessive insulin creates low blood sugar and so the craving for sugar continues.

Triglycerides

In 1958 Kinsall showed that the circulating saturated fats (triglycerides) were a main factor in clotting in heart attacks and not, as was suspected, the level of cholesterol. Of 100 patients who suffered heart attacks as a result of clots, only 18 per cent had blood cholesterol levels in excess of 250mg (normal range 120-300mg), while almost 90 per cent had an abnormally high level of triglycerides. It is interesting to learn that if a person with high blood fat level is under stress, the storage fat is released into the blood by the action of the adrenal hormones, and the blood fat levels can increase dramatically.

Ketosis

In a typical diet, half our energy is supplied from starch or sugar, the remaining half is provided by protein and fat. If we avoid carbohydrate completely and consume fat and protein only, our body uses stored carbohydrate (glycogen) as food. This supply is, however, used up within two to three days. After this time, the body fat is utilized and the main storage fat (triglyceride) is broken down into free fatty acids and 'ketones'. When fat is broken down in this way, so that the two fuels (fatty acids and ketones) are present in the blood, the process is known as *ketosis*. Many weight reducing diets are aimed at producing mild ketosis to burn off excessive fat. (Diabetics, however, can develop a more serious form of ketosis which can cause dangerous weight loss.) This controversial diet is called the ketogenic diet and is prescribed for a range of problems including hypoglycaemia, epilepsy and schizophrenia.

I have found in practice that a balanced wholefood diet, high in fresh fruit and vegetables and avoiding starch, is quite effective for reducing high levels of triglycerides and cholesterol in the blood. This is without insisting that patients avoid the cholesterol-rich foods (eggs, cheese, etc.) which are important sources of protein, vitamins, minerals and fats. Research has shown that to avoid cholesterol completely can be hazardous as it is an essential constituent of many hormones and assists the absorption of food. A low cholesterol diet can also have the unfortunate effect of stimulating the body to produce more cholesterol as only 20 per cent of our total cholesterol is provided by the food we eat. Unsaturated vegetable fats and phospholipids (lecithin) are of value in aiding utilization and transport of fat by clearing the fat deposited in the cells through the body. As we will see later when discussing treatment, this diet is virtually the same as the hypoglycaemic diet, and for this reason is of double value for the heart sufferer.

Mental Health

This covers a vast array of topics ranging from suicide and crime to schizophrenia, depression, anxiety and addictions. The mechanism whereby an inadequate supply of glucose to the brain cells can lead to personality disorders has been covered in previous chapters. It may, however, be of interest to delve a little deeper to show how poor nutrition and, in particular, low blood sugar, can affect the mind.

There is a tendency to attribute the great increase in mental illness over the last fifty years to the stressful effects of modern society. Sociologists and psychiatrists point to the damaging effects of television whereby the harrowing and distressing news from all over the world is introduced into our own homes. The economic pressures and competitiveness of society are blamed for the high incidence of anxiety neurosis, depression and nervous breakdowns. The consumption of tranquillizers and antidepressants is increasing year by year, and alcoholism and drug addiction is growing at an alarming rate. Antisocial behaviour and crimes of all types are also increasing. Can we really lay the blame for all this upon the pace of modern society? Surely there have been times in man's history when there was an equivalent or even greater degree of stress upon the individual? One has only to read Dickens, Zola or Tolstoy to appreciate the great despair and unhappiness that the majority of people experienced in previous centuries.

Do other, less advanced, cultures suffer the same mental problems as our own, and have the effects of stress in relation to nutrition ever been investigated in laboratory trials? Although there are no cut-and-dried answers to these questions, it may help to look a little closer at the history of stress in the hope that another explanation for the present epidemic of nervous ailments can be found.

Dr R. Williams, world famous chemist and nutritionist, wrote some years ago, 'The brain cells ultimately get from the blood only those nutrient elements that are furnished in the food we eat.[16] Perhaps, for many of us, this is an obvious statement, yet it is the work of Roger Williams, Linus Pauling and other nutritionists and researchers, who have paved the way for a more empirical explanation for mental disease, based not on altered personality and Freudian complexes, but on the biochemical requirements and nutritional imbalances within the brain and nervous system.

For many years it was assumed that vitamins, minerals and trace elements were needed by the body only in minute quantities, and that these quantities were adequately supplied by the normal Western diet. Roger Williams has, however, shown that individual requirements for certain substances vary enormously, and there are those who need ten to twenty times the average requirement of certain substances, just to maintain normal health. Dr Williams' book *Biochemical Individuality*[24] has caused a rethinking by the more enlightened health workers on the whole question of vitamin deficiency and the normal daily requirements of many substances. The book explains that many people suffer from mild vitamin deficiencies that give rise to personality disorders. This phenomenon is termed 'sub-clinical' as the more gross symptoms of pellagra, scurvy, rickets, etc. are not present. Dr Williams logically assumed that, between the so-called healthy individuals and those suffering from gross deficiency states, are many layers of mild deficiencies, often due not to deficient diets but to some individuals requiring huge amounts of vitamins not available in the typical diet. If we look at the symptoms of some of the vitamin deficient states (particularly Vitamin B), we can see that the *earliest* symptoms of deficiency usually involve the mind before physical symptoms show.

Vitamin B$_1$/Thiamine. The earliest deficiency symptoms include neurasthenia, depression, poor memory, fatigue, poor concentration, vague stomach and heart symptoms.

Vitamin B$_3$/Niacin, Nicotinic Acid, Nicotinamide. Earliest deficiency symptoms include neurasthenia, confusion, anxiety, fear, depression accompanied by skin, mouth and other ailments.

Vitamin C. Earliest symptoms of deficiency including bruising, poor healing, irritability, anxiety and depression.

Biotin. Earliest symptoms include fatigue, insomnia and anorexia.

Pantothenic Acid. Earliest deficiency symptoms include fatigue, apathy, depression, muscular weakness.

A great deal of research on animals and humans has confirmed that inadequate nutrition can have an effect upon the mind. Fortunately, in the early stages at least, these effects are reversible. In addition to depression and anxiety, actual personality changes have been recorded when subjects have agreed to follow vitamin-deficient diets, the old personality reappearing as the diet is normalized. Table 5 on page 65 gives a complete list of nutrients particularly relevant to mental health, and shows the variety of emotional conditions caused by a diet deficient in these nutrients.

Other factors influencing the effects of nutrition on the brain environment include drug side-effects, tobacco, alcohol, food additives, etc. When discussing nutrition to the brain, it should be remembered that the availability of adequate glucose to nerve tissue is essential for the efficient transport, absorption and utilization of many essential nutrients. Lewis showed in 1974[25] with animal tests that hypoglycaemia produced lethargy and weariness due to lowered absorption of essential brain nutrients. In the same journal, Lewis showed that hypoglycaemia can cause a decrease in the tissue concentration of most citric acid cycle (Krebs Cycle) components.[26] Vitamin B_1, pantothenic acid, Vitamin B_2 and B_3 are all closely involved with this cycle which is the 'major route of carbohydrate metabolism in the body[27] and is fundamental to our energy needs. It has also been shown that hypoglycaemia causes a decreased oxygen availability to brain tissue with resulting biochemical inefficiency.

Much work is still to be done on the connection between nutrition and the mind, but it is becoming clear that the role of blood sugar is vital for normal mental health.

Cancer

One person in every four in Europe and America will, at some time in his or her life, develop cancer. Although there are many different types of cancer, depending on location and tissue affected, there is growing evidence available to show a positive link between blood sugar levels and certain types of cancer.

The statistical evaluation of what, in America, is called D.D.D.'s (diabetes detection drives), when coupled with the patient's history of tumours, provided significant information which can be summarized as follows:

1. The risk of cancer increases as we get older.
2. People below 29 years reported no history of cancer.
3. Those in the 30-50 years age bracket with hypoglycaemia reported most cancer.

4. In the oldest age group, 50 and over, the incidence of cancer closely paralled the incidence of diabetes.

5. In all ages, overweight directly related to cancer incidence.

These susceptibility tests were carried out at the University of Alabama Medical Centre by Dr Cheraskin and Colleagues.[28] They concluded that the causes leading to hypoglycaemia and later, diabetes, were all contributive causes of cancer. It therefore follows that early detection and treatment of hypoglycaemia is one way to contribute to cancer prevention.

Alcoholism

It may seem out of place to include a section on alcoholism in a book on low blood sugar. There is, however, a strong connection between the two, and a reciprocal relationship exists between alcohol and blood sugar. Alcoholism can cause hypoglycaemia, and many experts accept that there is a condition known as alcohol-induced hypoglycaemia. Dr Tintera, an expert on alcoholism and blood sugar, has stated that, 'low blood sugar is central to the alcoholic problem'.

As described in Chapter 5, the symptoms of a hangover are due to hypoglycaemia. Unfortunately these symptoms are, for the alcoholic, chronic and recurring. The effect of alcohol is to lower the output of glucose by the liver, so triggering off or worsening existing hypoglycaemia. Conversely, the hypoglycaemic sufferer drinks because alcohol has the same effect as sugar.

In an interesting experiment, laboratory rats were divided into two groups. One group was provided with a high carbohydrate 'junk' diet, the other with a biologically ideal diet. Both groups were given a choice of water or alcohol to drink. The first group with the high sugar diet turned to the alcohol for drink, while their better-fed neighbours drank only water. These animals were not under stress, resentful, depressed, unhappy or frustrated. They just turned willingly to alcohol when their diet was inadequate. Furthermore, they became reformed alcoholics when their diets were improved and their carbohydrate level reduced.

In alcoholism a vicious circle develops with the alcohol providing a temporary uplift only to be followed by

Table 5. Effects of Nutritional Deficiencies on the Mind

Nutrient	Effects
Vitamin B_3 (niacin, nicotinic acid, nicotinamide) deficiency	Insomnia, nervousness, irritability, confusion, apprehensiveness, depression, hallucination.
Vitamin B_1 (thiamine) deficiency	Loss of appetite, depression, irritability, confusion, memory loss, inability to concentrate, sensitivity to noise.
Vitamin B_2 (riboflavin) deficiency	Depression.
Pantothenic acid deficiency	Depression, unable to tolerate stress.
Vitamin B_6 (pyridoxine) deficiency	Abnormal responses in psychotic children.
Vitamin B_{12} deficiency	Difficulty in concentration and remembering, stuporous depression, severe agitation, hallucinations, manic or paranoid behaviour.
Biotin deficiency	Depression, lassitude, panic, hallucinations.
Vitamin C administration	Improvement in schizophrenia.
Niacin supplement	Improvement in schizophrenia.
Iodine deficiency	Cretinism.
Potassium deficiency	Nervousness, irritability, mental disorientation.
Magnesium deficiency	Paranoid psychosis.
Threonine deficiency	Irritability, hard to get along with.
Lysine deficiency	Inability to concentrate.
Glutamic acid administration	Improvement in intelligence and general brain functioning in mental retardation.
Folic acid supplement	Improvement in psychosis.
Lactate excess in blood	Anxiety, neurosis, fatigue, insomnia, tension.
Calcium deficiency	Anxiety, neurosis, fatigue, insomnia, tension.

hypoglycaemia, until eventually only regular drinking achieves any comfort or relief. Alcoholics who succeed in drying out usually substitute sweets. They are still in a vicious circle, but perhaps a more socially acceptable one. Research has shown that the majority of alcoholics had a high sugar intake before their heavy drinking started, many craving sugar and sweet foods as children. The withdrawal symptoms of dry mouth, sweating and tremors experienced by the reformed alcoholics are, in part, due to an inability to correct their low blood sugar condition. This is aggravated by the habit of ex-alcoholics to eat sugar and chocolate when they experience these 'jitters'. Many reformed alcoholics who are, it is claimed, psychologically cured, have relapses owing to a continuing imbalance in their blood sugar. Simply to shift from alcohol to sugar is not the complete answer. The real answer once more lies in solving – through diet and other rational treatment – the underlying hypoglycaemia.

Drug Addiction
It is not a great step from alcoholism to drug addiction. Clinical studies by Dr Tintera have shown that alcoholics often become barbiturate addicts, and many heroin addicts have a positive glucose tolerance test result confirming hypoglycaemia. As with the alcoholic, the drug addict cannot usually afford good nutrition owing, in part, to the high cost of drugs, but also his abnormal craving for drugs replaces nutrition.

Many readers will be surprised to learn that there is a drug consumed on a daily basis by most of us which can cause great physical and emotional damage. That drug is caffeine.

Caffeinism
Also called 'coffee nerves', this condition has long been incorrectly thought of as psychological. Work by Dr J Greder,[29] Director of the Walker Reed U.S. Army Medical Centre, has shown that around 250mg of caffeine are sufficient to cause symptoms of caffeinism. These include shaking, headaches, anxiety, restlessness and lethargy. Table 6 shows the caffeine content of typical food, drinks and drugs. It will be seen that to consume 250mg would not be difficult or unusual. The figures are approximate.

Table 6. Caffeine Content of Typical Foods[30]

Food	Caffeine Content
Chocolate bar	160mg per 8oz (225g)
Aspirin-based tablets	15-30mg each
Coffee	100-150mg per cupful
Tea	60-75mg per cupful
Cola drinks	40-60mg per cupful

I have frequently encountered patients whose gross daily intake of caffeine is in excess of 1500mg.

Caffeine has an effect similar to sugar, although its action is not so immediate. It stimulates the adrenal glands to increase the blood sugar level, with a subsequent release of insulin to balance the sugar increase. For this reason, caffeine can act as a temporary stimulant to keep one awake. As with many other drugs, unpleasant withdrawal symptoms are experienced if the heavy coffee drinker attempts to stop the habit. Where there is a low tolerance of caffeine, anxiety and other emotional symptoms may be felt when consuming only two to three cups of coffee daily.

The addictive properties of caffeine in coffee have been investigated by many authorities. It has been demonstrated that coffee addicts show the recognizable signs of addiction. These are:

1. Able to tolerate coffee.
2. Unpleasant withdrawal symptoms when discontinuing.
3. A craving for coffee if deprived.

Caffeine produces a 'lift'. It creates a need in a similar way to alcohol, nicotine and a whole range of habit-forming substances. In the context of hypoglycaemia it constitutes a part cause and part effect. Just as alcohol, it becomes part of a vicious circle and, for this reason, caffeine, in the form of strong tea, coffee, chocolate or cola drinks, is totally banned from hypoglycaemic diets. I try to encourage patients to grow to like decaffeinated coffee and mild herbal teas.

Tobacco

By now you will be accusing me of being a killjoy. What is there left? Is nothing sacred? Nicotine creates a shock-wave in the blood sugar levels. Rises of 36-75 per cent in the blood glucose level have been shown in some studies. This is due to stimulation of the adrenal glands by the nicotine, rapidly followed by a drop in the glucose level. This see-saw effect explains the chain smoker's dilemma, for after each cigarette he craves another pick-up. Unfortunately, smoking creates a desire for caffeine, sweet foods and alcohol (smokers drink more often than non-smokers, indeed, the incidence of heavy drinking in smokers and non-smokers is in the proportion of two to one). The withdrawal symptoms are once more very similar to hypoglycaemic symptoms, i.e. headaches, drowsiness, trembling, anxiety and palpitations. Not surprisingly, smoking is a handicap in the treatment of hypoglycaemia, for often patients follow the correct diet but their symptoms do not change. There are two reasons for this:

1. Adrenal stimulation from nicotine constantly triggers the release of glucose into the blood.

2. Smoking is known to cause vitamin C loss. The rate of loss has been set at around 25mg per cigarette.[20] As this vitamin is connected with sugar metabolism controls, its value for the hypoglycaemic is indisputable.

There are obviously more serious health risks for the alcoholic, drug addict and heavy smoker than reactive hypoglycaemia. Owing to the reciprocal relationship of cause and effect with all these substances and hypoglycaemia, it can do nothing but good for the health of the 'user' to look to his or her nutrition to rebalance glucose levels and, with luck, 'kick the habit'.

Epilepsy

One of the many conditions that hypoglycaemia can mimic is epilepsy, also known as 'grand mal' or 'petit mal', depending on its severity. There are many types of epilepsy classified according to cause and symptoms. In the context of epilepsy due to hypoglycaemia I am referring chiefly to petit mal, the symptoms of which range from slight dizzy spells lasting several seconds to prolonged blackouts.

As long ago as the 1920s it was known that Islet tumours (tumours of the Islets of Langerhans – glands of the pancreas) caused convulsions and epileptic-type symptoms owing to insulin oversecretion. Removal of the tumours in most cases cured the patient of these symptoms. In 1947 Fabrykant noted that the E. E. G. patterns of epileptics were remarkably similar to those of the hypoglycaemic patients. For many years it has been known that epileptics tested with a six-hour glucose tolerance test often show a positive low blood sugar result.

Other clues are available to show the relationship between hypoglycaemia and epilepsy:

1. Pregnant epileptics often have fewer epileptic episodes or attacks, possibly owing to the higher blood sugar during pregnancy (see Chapter 8).

2. Many young epileptics have a craving for sweet foods and drinks, and the timing of epileptic attacks often coincides with the time when the blood sugar would be low, e.g. on rising and when meals are missed.

3. Stress, whether mental or physical (e.g. through taking coffee and sugar) have been known to trigger off an epileptic attack. As we know, stress also reduces the blood sugar level.

4. The diet usually prescribed for hypoglycaemics reduces epileptic symptoms.

Other factors are known to contribute to epileptic attacks, not least the role of calcium, magnesium and vitamin B_6 (pyridoxine). There seems little doubt, however, that when the complex process whereby glucose and its derivatives are made available to brain cells is thrown off balance by hypoglycaemia, epilepsy may be one of the results.

Stomach Ulcers

Reactive hypoglycaemia is thought to be partly caused by what is termed 'uncomplicated hyperinsulinism'. This is an excess of insulin in the blood due to an overactivity of the insulin apparatus. Although many glandular influences are involved, the end result is too much insulin and not enough sugar.

Studies have shown that hypoglycaemia causes a stimulus to the vagus nerve leading to increased secretion of gastric acids.[31] It is of interest to learn that the method of testing this reaction is to inject patients (animal and human) with intra-venous insulin. The German workers Feurle, Arnold, Eydt et al wrote in 1973 that: '. . . this rise in gastrin occurred fifteen minutes after the lowered blood sugar level had been reached and was accompanied by an abrupt rise in hydrochloric acid concentration.[32]

If we refer to a friend or colleague as 'a real ulcer case' we are referring to a certain type of stressful personality. It is generally accepted that severe mental and nervous stress can contribute to stomach ulcers. Dr Hans Seyle states examples of ulcers developing in a matter of days during the war before combat or after air raids.[15] The stomach wall becomes ulcerated owing to an inappropriate increase in stomach acid that is released either when no food is present in the stomach or is simply released in excessive quantities. In either case the stomach can literally digest itself.

The ulcer is perhaps the most common and obvious example of how the mind can affect the body. Unfortunately, the ulcer victim also suffers owing to the faulty breakdown in the absorption of food components, in particular protein, certain vitamins, calcium, etc. This tends to perpetuate his problems and his anxiety.

As with diabetes and asthma, the incidence of diabetic patients also having ulcers is very slight, and diabetics with ulcers who have been tested with a glucose tolerance test have been found to have dysinsulinism (fluctuating between high and low blood sugar). Abrahamson[17] tested 16 ulcer patients with a six-hour glucose tolerance test. All the patients had typical ulcer symptoms, i.e. heartburn and pain, etc. and the diagnosis of ulcers had been previously confirmed by x-ray findings. All the 16 showed conclusive signs of hypoglycaemia.

Because there are so many interrelated factors when considering the cause of ulcers, it is not possible to say that hypoglycaemia is the sole cause. Many ulcer patients do not exhibit the typical hypoglycaemic symptoms. It seems likely, however, that by the same token stress is not the sole cause and is invariably accompanied by dietary considerations. The intake of protein, coffee, nicotine, vitamins and many drugs all affect the stomach acid. If stress alone is the cause of ulcers, why was the incidence of stomach ulcers higher in American training camps in World War Two than in the actual fighting units in combat conditions? Abrahamson believes this paradox is due to the greater consumption of caffeine contained in soft drinks and coffee in the training camps. The high-starch Western diet has resulted in a hugh increase in the incidence of stomach ulcers. Dr Cleave states in his book *The Peptic Ulcer*[33] that the incidence of peptic ulcers parallels the intake of refined starches. He believes that over several million years of evolution man has learned how to deal with stress and, for this reason, it is not a causative factor in ulcer production.

Perhaps the answer lies somewhere between the nutrition and the stress schools of thought. Once more in the hypoglycaemia story we are presented with a vicious circle – incorrect diet and stress leading to hypoglycaemia which leads to further stress and dietary imbalance owing to the ulcer symptoms. The circle is complete.

The treatment of the ulcer patient is very similar to the many other conditions caused by hypoglycaemia, and the stressful symptoms that contribute to the problem are often also relieved.

Obesity

Hypoglycaemia has been called the 'hunger disease'. The fluctuations in blood sugar levels cause frequent hunger pangs that are relieved only by constantly overeating. The inevitable consequence of this is becoming overweight, for unless the consumption of carbohydrates is balanced by a very high energy output (as in the case of the athlete or the labourer), the excess carbohydrate is converted to glycogen and stored in the liver and muscles. We know that hypoglycaemia, whether expressed as alcoholism, stomach ulcers or anxiety neurosis, is invariably temporarily relieved by taking more sugar. For this reason there is a close relationship between overweight and hypoglycaemia. It has been estimated that 20 per cent of the population are overweight. The obese person who 'must' have a chocolate, the alcoholic who 'must' have one more drink, are probably suffering from the same withdrawal symptoms brought about by low blood sugar.

Insulin is the only hormone in the body that promotes the storage of fuel. For this reason it is often termed the 'fattening hormone'. It converts and stores carbohydrate to glycogen and fat to triglyceride. So hypoglycaemia promotes fat and overweight in two ways:

1. The excessive insulin invariably found in hypoglycaemia causes the body to deposit fat in the tissues.
2. Hypoglycaemia increases hunger and sugar craving.

Except for thyroid imbalance and certain rare metabolic defects, overweight is caused by overeating. The problem in the overweight person is not one of what to eat and what diet to follow; the calorie-controlled or carbohydrate unit-controlled diets are readily available. The problem lies in self-control in overcoming the almost overpowering craving to eat. Unfortunately for the hypoglycaemic, the urge is to eat high sugar foods that cause more weight increase. It is essential, however, that the overweight patient considers every aspect of weight control: simply to follow a 500-600 calorie diet could be disastrous. Thyroid output may need to be checked and the effects of fluid retention due to a variety of causes should not be overlooked.

Hypoglycaemia leads to stress with subsequent potassium loss and sodium retention. This causes a waterlogging of tissues known as oedema. For many reasons, simply to reduce food intake is not always the answer. What is often required is an interim period to resolve the blood sugar imbalance, thyroid imbalance or fluid imbalance before dieting commences. If your weight is not reduced by a 1000-calories-a-day diet then advice should be sought on the many possible reasons for overweight.

It is generally accepted that overweight is an adverse complication in many conditions relating to hypoglycaemia, including osteo-arthritis, heart disease and diabetes.

Neuralgia

As you may recall from previous discussion, hypoglycaemia can cause swelling and pressure around blood vessels due to vasodilation. This compensatory mechanism can lead to headaches, particularly migraine. I have observed, however, that another equally stubborn condition can be caused or aggravated by hypoglycaemia, that is trigeminal neuralgia – or tic douloureux. The trigeminal nerve is one of a group of twelve nerves known as the cranial nerves. It branches into three nerves, which in turn pass to the forehead and the eye region, the cheek and the jaw. The neuralgia can involve any combination of these three nerves and can be, at times, very severe and resistant to treatment. Trigeminal sufferers frequently experience an aggravation of their symptoms shortly after eating sweet foods, in a similar way to the migraine sufferers. I have therefore found that diet along the lines of the hypoglycaemia diet has often proved of benefit.

Quite apart from the possible local pressure due to vasodilation (as in migraine) hypoglycaemia can cause calcium reduction in the blood, creating a general irritability of the nervous system (see Chapter 7). This would no doubt contribute to neuralgia symptoms anywhere in the body.

Fatigue

One of the most common symptoms occurring in hypoglycaemia is fatigue. Glucose and its derivatives provide fuel to the nerve cells. It follows, therefore, that if the fuel is in short supply, the available energy must be reduced. Exhaustion is difficult to treat because there are so many causes. These include:

1. *Stress.* Stress can be likened to a stationary car. If you apply the choke or put your foot on the throttle the engine increases revs and uses fuel, but it does not move. In a like manner, the stressful individual may exhaust himself by simply sitting and worrying. Stress causes the adrenal glands to operate the 'fight or flight' mechanism. This may be very necessary in primitive, natural environments, but can be destructive and fatiguing on a daily basis, as often occurs in civilized society.

2. *Overwork.* I am often amazed at the number of hours a day many people work, although this particularly applies to the self-employed, but also there are many who 'moonlight', e.g. they have two jobs involving a twelve to sixteen hour day. Unfortunately, those who work hard and long often miss holidays and have erratic meal times. Not surprisingly their body cannot stand the pace and fatigue develops.

3. *Insomnia.* When confronted with a patient with fatigue, the first question must be 'Do you sleep well?' Insufficient sleep night after night, for whatever reason, must lead to extreme fatigue. Even when the diet is perfect and there is no undue stress, insufficient sleep is a prime cause of fatigue. Individual sleep requirements vary enormously – some of us can manage with five hours, others may even need nine or ten hours.

4. *Smoking and drinking.* There is little need to repeat what has been said in previous chapters as both habits are destructive and energy-sapping. Faulty nutrition and low blood sugar are one of the main causes of fatigue. Nutritional deficiencies and deficiency of the blood itself can contribute to low energy.

Dr Williams has found that fatigue can result from individual requirements for vitamins and minerals far in excess of accepted normal requirements.[24] If these requirements are not met with supplements to the diet, then that person may become extremely tired. There is no quick answer to the person who is constantly tired. Elimination of the foregoing list is perhaps a first step to solving the problem. It should be remembered, however, that fatigue is a symptom of many serious illnesses requiring detailed and specific tests, and these include:

Diabetes	Leukaemia
Arthritis	Acute and chronic infections
Cancer	Drug side effects
Anaemia	Nervous disorders
Thyroid imbalance	Absorption problems
Heart conditions	T.B.
Malnutrition	Kidney disease

This chapter has, I hope, shown the diversity of diseases and symptoms that can be caused or influenced by hypoglycaemia. All the conditions discussed can be due to other causes. It is worth remembering, however, that there is, in every instance, a link with hypoglycaemia which has been proved, and evidence is available to show that the dietary approach so essential in hypoglycaemia has provided symptom relief – often in many cases where other treatment has failed.

10

DIAGNOSIS

As hypoglycaemia masquerades as so many different conditions and can create such a diversity of symptoms, it is not always easy to diagnose. For this reason, and others which will be discussed later, it is not wise to diagnose and treat hypoglycaemia without professional help. Hypoglycaemia mimics very many serious diseases, and it is therefore essential that the more serious causes of hypoglycaemic symptoms be ruled out.

The clinical diagnosis of hypoglycaemia falls into several stages.

Family History

Although this subject has been briefly touched upon in other parts of the book, I would like to show, with examples, just how hypoglycaemic conditions can pass from generation to generation. It follows that detailed information of a person's family health is of considerable diagnostic value.

In Table 1 you will see the family history of 50 patients with confirmed reactive hypoglycaemia (as proved by a six-hour glucose tolerance test). These have been selected as typical low blood sugar problems and you will see that the characteristic symptoms associated with hypoglycaemia pass through each family. The majority of patients with a positive glucose tolerance test result tend to show a previous history in their family of either asthma, migraine, hay fever, diabetes, epilepsy or depression, etc.

Present Symptoms

As we know, the symptoms of hypoglycaemia can be misleading to the diagnostician: often of more significance than a list of symptoms is the pattern of cause and the time of onset of the symptoms. One patient, Mr A, may experience headaches when reading or watching television, while another patient, Mr B, may develop headaches only in the early morning or when he drinks certain types of wine. In the case of Mr A, he may well have eye strain, but Mr B could be a subject for hypoglycaemia.

Fatigue at the end of the day may suggest overwork, anaemia or a variety of causes. Fatigue on rising which improves towards the end of the day is a strong clue to a possible diagnosis of hypoglycaemia. A subjective evaluation is never easy, for unless one is very familiar with the pattern of hypoglycaemic symptoms, it is very difficult to diagnose one's own problem.

One of the chief characteristics of hypoglycaemia sufferers is the combination of physical and mental symptoms coupled with considerable variation in the symptoms. At times the patient may feel on top of the world, and at other times he may feel exhausted and depressed for no apparent reason. Remember, we are not dealing with a predictable organic disease such as overactive thyroid or anaemia, but an imbalance in the nervous, circulatory, digestive and endocrine systems. Therefore, any symptoms are the expression of a great number of interrelating and fluctuating factors. These factors are influenced by diet, emotion, menstruation, time of day, stress and fatigue, and other factors already mentioned.

Past Health
No illness suddenly arrives. There are always changes in the body before the symptoms become apparent to the patient. With hypoglycaemia the early symptoms are usually vague and difficult to identify. The commonest symptoms are fatigue associated with a dulling of concentration, irritability and mild anxiety or depression, thick-headedness on wakening and a distinct loss of zest before mid-morning. The latter symptoms may include transitory feelings of panic or breathlessness with cold sweating and headaches often accompanied by a craving for something sweet. These early symptoms are often diagnosed as being due to overwork, stress or nerves. The usual sedatives and relaxants are prescribed, but if symptoms are due to hypoglycaemia any relief will be only temporary. The fatigue will still be there and often without overwork, and the anxiety will persist often without any known

stress. It is unfortunate that many hypoglycaemic patients suffer their symptoms with a false diagnosis, for years classified by doctors and family as neurotic when, in fact, the cause of their symptoms is physiological and not psychological.

When looking into a past health history, there is often a history of symptoms that show promise of future hypoglycaemia. These include hepatitis, jaundice, morning sickness with pregnancy, biliousness and intolerance of fats, and a history of gall bladder trouble. The role of the body's early warning system is to indicate the development of a biochemical imbalance or damage of some kind. If the early symptoms of hypoglycaemia are accurately diagnosed before the migraines, epilepsies and diabetes develop, a great deal of pain and distress may be avoided.

Dietary Habits

Faulty nutrition can be said to be the single most important cause of hypoglycaemia. The modern diet with its high sugar content, refined starches, artificial additives, and with taste and appearance taking commercial priority over nutritional value, is the perfect combination for causing blood sugar imbalances. If we also consider the modern habits of snack-meals, frequent coffees and the excessive use of drugs, alcohol and tobacco, it is no surprise that the incidence of high and low blood sugar conditions is increasing at an alarming rate.

As poor diet is a key factor in the cause and maintenance of hypoglycaemia, it is obviously an important clue in the diagnosis of this problem. I find in practice that most hypoglycaemic sufferers have characteristic dietary habits which provide an important clue to the cause of their symptoms. It must be remembered that, for the hypoglycaemic, meals are not simply a question of choice, for the pattern of meals and type of food is strongly influenced by the underlying low blood sugar. Sugary foods and drink, caffeine-rich or alcohol-rich drinks all provide temporary relief to the symptoms of hypoglycaemia. Not surprisingly, the diet reflects this and is high in these items. Often there may be cravings for sweet food, etc. far in excess of normal consumption and, as discussed in Chapter 9, most alcoholics and tobacco addicts are hypoglycaemic.

One of the most significant clues is the sugar intake – two to three teaspoonsful in either tea or coffee is not unusual.

Because hypoglycaemia is linked to the appetite, a frequent symptom is hunger; not the type of hunger that most of us experience if we miss a meal, but a ravenous hunger, very often a craving for a certain type of food. Conversely, the hypoglycaemic patient, because of the symptoms produced by his condition, cannot face food. This usually occurs at breakfast time as the blood sugar drops overnight. The thought of breakfast can make a person with hypoglycaemia almost physically sick. Usually a coffee or cigarette starts the day, and the inevitable 'high' provided by the caffeine produces a mid-morning 'low' as the blood sugar drops again. So the day consists of small frequent 'shots' of sugar or caffeine to keep the energy level and the concentration in a tolerable balance.

The hypoglycaemic is a night nibbler, often waking with stomach cramp, indigestion or just hunger, usually around 3 a.m. to 5 a.m. when the blood sugar has sunk to a low level.

The two diets listed below are not only typical diets of those who become hypoglycaemic, but the the actual diets of two patients seen in my practice. Every characteristic of the hypoglycaemic's eating habits can be seen here and, although in each case a glucose tolerance test was requested, the two patients were inevitably hypoglycaemic.

Example 1

Breakfast: Cereal with sugar and milk. 4-5 cups of tea – 1 teaspoonful of sugar in each cup.

11 a.m.   Tea with a biscuit or cake.

Lunch: Sandwich with tea and biscuit.

4 p.m.:   Cake with tea.

Dinner: Meat and vegetables with sweet dessert. Cup of tea.

Supper: Crackers, cheese, biscuits and tea.

— Tea – 12-14 cups daily.
— Coffee – rarely.
— Cigarettes – 20-30 a day.
— Sweets and chocolate – 4-6oz (100-175g) a day.

Example 2

Breakfast: 2 coffees with 2½ teaspoonsful of sugar in each.

11 a.m.:   Coffee with biscuits.

Lunch: Toast with egg on cheese. 2 coffees.

4.30 p.m.: Cake with coffee.
Dinner: Meat and vegetables with coffee.
Supper: Cake with coffee.

— Tea – nil.
— Coffee – 8-10 cups daily.
— Cigarettes – 10-12 a day.
— Sweets and chocolate – 2oz (50g) a day approximately.

Physical Examination

There is only one physical sign of hypoglycaemia – a tenderness above the pancreas in the left upper quadrant of the abdomen, often extending as low as the umbilicus. This tenderness is felt just below the rib, or at times round the side of the rib cage. It is due to pancreatic sensitivity which, as we know, is due to hyperinsulinism. In practice I find that if I press most patients' abdomens hard enough they are tender in many places. The test is therefore to press with the same gentle pressure all over the stomach, liver and pancreas areas and then ask the patient, 'Which is the most tender?' The fingers encounter a feeling of tightness, or even hardness, accompanying the discomfort. This sign usually disappears as treatment progresses, and provides confirmation that the situation is normalizing.

Although the patient's weight, colouring, blood pressure, etc. are all significant in hypoglycaemia, they are all influenced by many other disorders and are therefore not of particular value in diagnosing hypoglycaemia.

The Six-hour Glucose Tolerance Test

This test is the most reliable test for reactive hypoglycaemia and is usually referred to as the G.T.T. The customary test of two hours is frequently used, and although it may be sufficient for a diagnosis of diabetes, it is virtually valueless as a means of establishing reactive hypoglycaemia, since the important overswing invariably occurs after more than two hours. The G.T.T. is only a valid diagnostic tool if the following conditions are met:

1. It is combined with a physical examination.
2. The test is preceded by noting down a detailed case history.
3. The patient has described and listed his own diet and symptoms.

4. The patient's reactions and symptoms during the test are noted and timed.
5. The glucose dosage and timing of blood sample taking is standardized for every test.
6. No dramatic changes have recently been made to the diet.
7. The physician is fully aware of any drugs being taken by the patient.

It must be remembered that some hypoglycaemics do not show symptoms, while other patients show pronounced hypoglycaemic symptoms with a normal blood sugar level. Hence the need to standardize the test procedures and to know each patient as thoroughly as possible before the test.

Test Procedure
The patient is requested to undergo a twelve-hour fast, (water only permitted), and to attend the surgery at 9.00 a.m. The fast is no great hardship as only breakfast is missed. Obviously it is important that no food or drink (except water) is taken until the test is completed at 3.30 p.m.

During the course of the test, seven small blood samples are taken from the veins of the arm. (Only 1 ml of whole blood being required per sample.) The first sample, taken at 9.15 a.m., shows the level of fasting blood sugar (F.B.S.), and is followed at 9.30 a.m. by the drinking of 50g (2oz) of soluble glucose. The remaining six samples are then taken to monitor the effects of the glucose on the patient's blood sugar level. The amount of glucose used in the G.T.T. can vary, 100g (4oz) being the usual test dose in America. This higher dose can occasionally make the more sensitive patients nauseous or faint, and is not normally used in this country. (There is no available evidence to suggest that 100g (4oz) improves diagnostic accuracy.)

The blood sugar level is constantly changing and, even with seven samples taken in six hours, one obtains only a guide to the dynamics of blood glucose activities. For this reason, the highest reading may in fact lie *between* two samples. If I suspect that this has occurred and the speed of the patient's insulin response has been so rapid that the G.T.T. has not confirmed diagnosis – a repeat test is requested. This is a shorter version, also using 50g (2oz) of glucose but with a sample taken every

15 minutes over a 1½-hour period. In this way the all-important upper figure is more precisely assessed.

The sample times are obviously at the convenience of the practitioner. I find the following schedule most suitable.

Patient arrives — — — — — — — — — — 9.00 a.m.
Sample 1. F.B.S. taken — — — — — — — 9.15 a.m.
50g glucose taken— — — — — — — — — 9.30 a.m.
Sample 2.— — — — — — — — — — — — 10.00 a.m.
Sample 3.— — — — — — — — — — — — 10.30 a.m.
Sample 4.— — — — — — — — — — — — 11.30 a.m.
Sample 5.— — — — — — — — — — — — 12.30 a.m.
Sample 6.— — — — — — — — — — — — 2.00 p.m.
Sample 7.— — — — — — — — — — — — 3.30 p.m.

This means that the samples are taken at the following times *after* drinking the glucose.

Sample 2.— — — — — — — — — — — — ½ hour
Sample 3.— — — — — — — — — — — — 1 hour
Sample 4.— — — — — — — — — — — — 2 hours
Sample 5.— — — — — — — — — — — — 3 hours
Sample 6.— — — — — — — — — — — — 4½ hours
Sample 7.— — — — — — — — — — — — 6 hours

The patient is encouraged to keep active during the tests, keeping, if possible, within his own normal daily energy output, and is required at the surgery only for the sample-taking. (If symptoms develop during the second half of the test a restroom is available when needed.)

As many patients do not feel very alert after the completion of the test, they are advised to arrange for a 'chauffeur' (relative or neighbour) to drive them home. It is also sensible to have some bread and cheese or a glass of milk as soon as possible after the test is completed.

Symptoms Produced by the G.T.T.
The symptoms that arise during the test, and the timing of the onset of these symptoms are both of considerable diagnostic value.

When the glucose readings are explained to the patient on his/her next visit, it is always interesting to note that the symptoms experienced during the test, (e.g. nausea, headache, stomach pains, lethargy, dizziness), usually arise as the blood sugar falls. The majority of patients are quite impressed to learn that their symptoms often attributed to stress or imagination can be reproduced by the simple method of taking a glucose drink. For them, this confirms the diagnosis of hypoglycaemia in a far more tangible way than could a set of blood test results. This clinical confirmation of a puzzling condition is often very reassuring to the patient.

G.T.T. Results

This valuable test can establish a diagnosis of diabetes or hypoglycaemia. Although the medical orthodox view holds that reactive hypoglycaemia is a rare condition, the evidence points to the contrary. I have found that out of 210 patients selected and tested with a six-hour G.T.T., 92% showed clearly defined reactive hypoglycaemia.

Since Seale Harris first described hypoglycaemia in 1924, no one generally accepted guideline defining this condition has been agreed upon. The G.T.T. is open to various interpretations, depending on the doctor's view of what constitutes the 'normal'. (As with many types of measurement used in medicine, the figures for the average patient cannot necessarily be taken as the normal!)

Dr Harris has stated, that in his view a diagnosis of hypoglycaemia is justified if the G.T.T. shows a blood sugar reading *below* the commonly accepted lower limit (70-100mg/ 100ml). This, he insisted, must be supported by the reproduction of hypoglycaemic symptoms during the course of the test. Over the intervening years the required lower limit, below which hypoglycaemia could be established, has been reduced to 40mg/100ml.

This rather rigid criterion for diagnosis has fortunately been modified in recent years, with the general recognition that each G.T.T. result should be assessed in relation to the patient. An individual's response to the glucose drink should be observed in terms of speed of absorption, and speed of insulin response.

A patient may have pronounced symptoms of hypoglycaemia yet show a set of glucose readings, all of which are within 'normal' limits. Close attention to symptoms before and during the G.T.T. is of greater diagnostic value than slavish adherence to a set of normal ranges.

I have seen patients experience distressing symptoms of hypoglycaemia when their blood sugar has fallen during a G.T.T. from 140mg to 70mg, the symptoms being caused not by the *level* of glucose but by the inappropriate *speed* of the fall.

It may be of value to discuss the *normal* G.T.T. result, before going further, and the manner in which the result is presented.

Table 7. Normal Six-hour G.T.T. Result

Sample	Interval from 0 in hours	Time	Result in mg/100ml
1	0 (F.B.S.)	9.15 a.m.	80
	(50g glucose solution)	(9.30 a.m.)	
2	½	10.00 a.m.	140
3	1	10.30 a.m.	130
4	2	11.30 a.m.	85
5	3	12.30 p.m.	73
6	4½	2.00 p.m.	75
7	6	3.30 p.m.	80

When the glucose has been taken by the patient, the blood sugar rises (Samples 2 and 3). As the glucose is absorbed, insulin is automatically released to control the rising blood sugar. With a normal insulin response, only an optimum amount of insulin is released allowing the blood sugar level to fall to the patient's fasting level (Sample 7).

The results are plotted on a graph and a glucose tolerance curve is produced. Examples of typical curves are shown below (Figures 5-14). One learns to recognize different types of curves, for the configuration of a curve is diagnostically as important as the actual figures producing it.

Diagnosis Using the G.T.T.

When presented with a set of figures for a G.T.T. the first step is to look for a possible diabetic component. A fasting level in excess of 120mg/100ml is strongly suggestive of diabetes, but some diabetics can have a fasting level under 100mg/100ml. For this reason an assessment of the sum of the first four results obtained in the G.T.T. is recommended by Dr Danowski of Pittsburg,[20] as a more reliable method of identifying diabetes. If the *total* for the four samples is between 500 and

800, diabetes is suspected; if *over* 800, diabetes is positively confirmed.

There are many different types of G.T.T. curves, for the dynamics of the blood sugar level is expressed in many ways. As stated, the actual level of blood sugar is related to symptoms during the test, but even more important is, perhaps, the speed at which the blood sugar responds to the insulin. A drop of from 120mg to 60mg in one hour may be more significant than a drop from 120mg to 40mg in two hours. The time taken for the sugar to return to a normal level (usually called the 'recovery'), and how long it remains at a low level, are also important diagnostic clues. For example, a fall to 40mg with a rapid recovery to normal may be less significant than a fall to 60mg that stays at this level for two to three hours before recovery.

It is very unusual to find any two G.T.T. curves that are alike. So called 'normal' values are based on population averages and may not reflect what is normal for the patient being tested.

Some disagreement surrounds the value of interpreting the 'fall' in blood sugar during the test. This represents the difference between the initial fasting level, and the lowest figure to which the blood sugar drops during the test. Atkins[20] considers a 30mg drop essential before a conclusive diagnosis of hypoglycaemia can be given, whilst Fredericks[34] finds that a drop of between 10-20mg is sufficient. Other authorities (e.g. Somgyi) have set the figures of 3-5mg as diagnostically significant. These figures are, however, meaningful only within the context of symptoms arising during the test and an individual's reaction to the 50g (2oz) of glucose. I find in practice that as little as a 5mg fall can be associated with hypoglycaemic symptoms.

To conclude this description of the G.T.T., it may be worth quoting Carlton Fredericks,[34] an authority on many aspects of nutrition. He states that 'when blood sugar drops as little as 2mg below the *normal for the patient*, a profound glandular compensation may start'.

In his view, no practitioner should disregard a blood sugar reading that is 'only a few points below normal' and if there is doubt, a diagnosis of hypoglycaemia with correct treatment should be considered.

Below are some typical blood sugar curves.

Figure 5. Normal blood sugar curves.

Normal Blood Sugar Curves

These curves are of healthy individuals. The fasting test (the first reading) varies, but at no time during the six hours does the blood sugar fall much below the fasting level.

Figure 6. Flat sugar-tolerance fatigue curve.

Flat Sugar-tolerance 'Fatigue' Curve

This type of curve can be seen as a modified form of hypoglycaemia. The patient's absorption of glucose is poor and the level does not fall or rise. This result reflects a fatigued, depressed individual.

Figure 7. Mild pre-hypoglycaemic curve (slow descent).

Mild, Pre-hypoglycaemic Curve

After the third hour, the blood sugar level drops below the fasting level, as the insulin builds up in the blood. Even after six hours the level of blood sugar has not returned to the patient's normal (fasting) level.

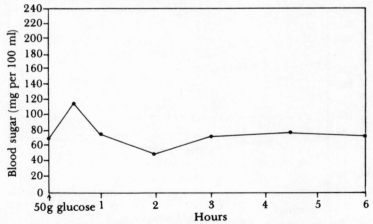

Figure 8. Mild pre-hypoglycaemic curve (rapid descent).

Mild Hypoglycaemia

Although there is not a great difference between the fasting level and the lowest point reached, the *speed* of descent suggests rapid and excessive insulin reaction.

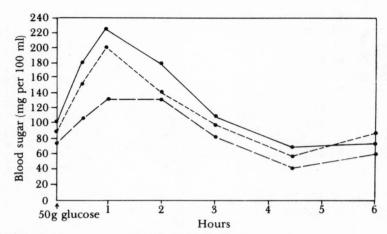

Figure 9. Reactive hypoglycaemia (typical curves).

Reactive Hypoglycaemia (Typical Curves)
All the signs of true reactive hypoglycaemia can be seen here.
The rapid absorption and rise in blood sugar; followed by the
hypoglycaemic 'low' point reached after four hours, and the
partial recovery by the six-hour test.

Figure 10. Reactive hypoglycaemia showing after three hours
(typical curves).

Reactive Hypoglycaemia, Showing After Three Hours
A common result, emphasizing the limitations of the two or
three hour G.T.T. Note that the severe hypoglycaemia only
shows itself after three hours; the early part of the test being
quite normal.

Figure 11. Reactive hypoglycaemia (severe curves).

Reactive Hypoglycaemia (Severe Curves)

Often a low fasting level with a further drop into very low readings. Patients with symptoms during the test are usually found to have this type of severe curve.

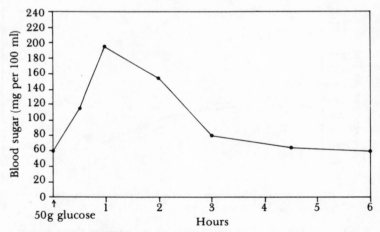

Figure 12. Pre-diabetic curve.

Pre-Diabetic Curve

Steep rise in blood sugar with very slow return to normal level. Characteristics of sluggish pre-diabetic insulin response.

Figure 13. Dysinsulinism

Dysinsulinism

The blood sugar paradox. Delayed insulin response causing high blood sugar, with an appropriate insulin excess in the third hour, causing hypoglycaemic-type fall.

Figure 14. Diabetic curve.

Diabetic Curve

Typical diabetic curves, high fasting levels and insufficient insulin to normalize blood sugar level.

11

THE TREATMENT OF HYPOGLYCAEMIA

I wish that I could state that there is *one* diet recommended by the various 'experts' for treating reactive hypoglycaemia. Regrettably this is not the case, as most of the writers and specialists seem to want to promote their own diet. This should seem to offer a welcome variety to the reader and choice to the patient; unfortunately, it causes only confusion. This occurs mainly because of the common habit of most writers on hypoglycaemia of recommending their own treatment programme at the expense of other treatments, frequently stating that the other people's diets and treatment are useless or even dangerous.

Dietary Requirements
There are, however, certain principles or requirements which must be met if a diet for hypoglycaemia is to be effective. These can be listed as follows:

1. Total carbohydrate consumption must be reduced, and refined (quickly absorbed) carbohydrates, including sugar, chocolates, sweets etc. must be *avoided*.

2. There should be five or six small meals daily.

3. The diet should be relatively high in fat and protein which should be spread over the day.

4. The total calorie content of the diet should be around 2,500 calories.

5. The diet should include a substantial breakfast and supper, to be taken as early and as late as possible.

6. Stimulants that will increase and subsequently lower the blood sugar (owing to hyperinsulinism) must be avoided. These include alcohol, tobacco and excessive exercise.

Although I do not agree with some of the diets recommended by American authors, it may be of interest to discuss briefly the various dietary approaches to hypoglycaemia. (One problem with reading too many American publications on hypoglycaemia is that the American diet is somewhat different from the English diet. We rarely come across egg plant, kohlrabi or collards on a British shopping list!)

The Seale Harris Diet (High Fat and High Protein)
Still recommended by many doctors and writers, this diet was described by Dr Harris in his first paper on hypoglycaemia,[8] and has a strong supporter in Dr Abrahamson.[17]
The Harris diet is as follows:

On rising:	100ml (4 fl oz) of orange juice.
Breakfast:	1 fruit, with or without cream – no sugar. 1 serving of cereal with cream – no sugar. 1 egg and, if desired, 2 or 3 slices of bacon. 1 slice of bread or toast with butter (liberally spread). Caffeine-free coffee, or very weak tea – no sugar.
2 hours after breakfast:	75ml (3 fl oz) of orange juice or 100ml (4 fl oz) of tomato juice.
3 hours after breakfast:	1 glass of milk.
Dinner:	Soup (cold or jellied chicken or beef *consommé*) or tomato juice. 225g (8oz) vegetables. 1 large portion of meat, poultry or fish. 1 slice of bread or toast. Fruit with cream.

3 hours after dinner:	1 glass of milk.
1 hour before supper:	75 ml (3 fl oz) of orange juice or 100 ml (4 fl oz) of tomato juice.
Supper:	One meat 'substitute' – egg, cheese or fish. Salad – large serving of lettuce, cole slaw, tomato or Waldorf salad with mayonnaise or french dressing. 1 portion of vegetables. 1 slice of bread with plenty of butter. Fruit.
2-3 hours after supper:	1 glass of milk.
Every 2 hours until bed-time:	100 ml (4 fl oz) of orange or tomato juice.

It has been used as a basis for many of the diets prescribed for hypoglycaemia, and we owe a great deal to Dr Harris for his observations almost sixty years ago.

The Airola Diet
(Low Animal Protein – High Natural Carbohydrate)
The American author, Dr Paavo Airola, has evolved a diet that contains (in order of importance):

1. Grains, seeds and nuts
2. Vegetables
3. Fruit

Dr Airola claims that raw and sprouted grains and seeds should be the main protein source, animal proteins being kept to a minimum. All seeds and nuts are eaten fresh and raw, and cereals are permitted provided they are eaten in their 'whole' state and not refined. Millet is especially recommended. He recommends that meat be eaten on a weekly basis, if at all. The diet is as follows:

7 a.m.	Glass of fruit juice. Sweet juices must be diluted with water 50/50.

8 a.m.   BREAKFAST. Nuts, seeds, fruit, yogurt, cottage cheese,
                OR, cooked cereal with oil and raw milk.

10 a.m.   Snack – a few nuts, or glass of yogurt, or piece of fruit.

12 noon   Glass of fresh juice.

1 p.m.   LUNCH. Cooked cereal: buckwheat, millet, etc. with oil and milk, if not not eaten for breakfast, OR, fruit or vegetable salad with yogurt and 2 slices of wholewheat bread with cheese and butter.

3 p.m.   Glass of juice or kefir with 2 tablespoonsful of yeast.

5 p.m.   Glass of fresh vegetable juice.

6 p.m.   DINNER. Vegetable salad with cooked vegetable dish of: beans, tortillas, yams, green beans, baked potatoes, etc. Slice or two of wholewheat bread. Cottage cheese, yogurt. Animal protein if desired.

8 p.m.   Glass of milk or yogurt with 1 or 2 tablespoonsful of brewer's yeast.

High Protein Diet
Perhaps the commonest dietary treatment of hypoglycaemia is simply to instruct patients to avoid all forms of refined starch and eat lots of protein and fat. Fredericks advocates a daily consumption of 300-375g(11-13oz) of meat. This should be in the form of six meals with meat or 'meat substitute' (e.g. cheese) at every meal.

Common Factors
Clearly these various diets for hypoglycaemia are all quite different; yet in each case the diet seems to work, and evidence is available to confirm the efficiency of each regime. This paradox is probably due to certain common factors in the diets, namely, the avoidance of refined starch and the insistence upon five or six regular meals.

Diets work only if the patient is prepared to follow them for a prescribed period of time. With the hypoglycaemic diet it is essential to maintain the diet for an initial period of eight to twelve weeks. It follows that any diet must fulfil these requirements:

1. It should not contain expensive or exotic food (e.g. fillet steak daily).
2. Many patients work full time and cannot prepare elaborate dishes; the meals must be simple, particularly as there are four to six meals per day.
3. The diet should not be too unsociable and too different from the average diet. Otherwise, I have found that patients are too easily tempted to 'stray' off the recommended foods.
4. The meals should be tasty and enjoyable.
5. Since many hypoglycaemics are overweight (especially the ladies), and very conscious of extra pounds, the diet should not cause one to put on weight.
6. Finally, and perhaps most obvious, the diet must work. Only by feeling better will a patient continue to follow a strict diet, week after week.

It is quite impossible to draw up an individual diet for each patient. I use, therefore, a standard diet for hypoglycaemia and encourage patients to talk over any problems or uncertainties.

Recommended Diet
The standard diet that I use is as follows:

On rising: Medium orange, ½ grapefruit or 100ml (4 fl oz) fruit juice or cup of beverage or milk.

Breakfast: Fruit or 100ml (4 fl oz) fruit juice.
                1 egg, with or without 2 slices of ham or bacon.
                1 slice of wholewheat bread or toast, with plenty of butter.
                Milk or beverage.

2 hours after   100ml (4 fl oz) fruit juice.
breakfast:

Lunch:	Meat, fish, cheese or eggs with salad – large serving of lettuce or tomato with mayonnaise or french dressing. Vegetables if desired. 1 slice of wholewheat bread, toast or crispbread with plenty of butter.
3 hours after lunch:	100ml (4 fl oz) milk.
1 hour before dinner:	100ml (4 fl oz) fruit juice.
Dinner:	Soup, if desired (not thickened with flour). Vegetables. Meat, fish or poultry. 1 slice of wholewheat bread, if desired. Dessert (fruit – fresh, stewed or baked) and beverage.
Every 2 hours until bed-time:	Small handful of nuts (unsalted).
Supper:	Crispbread with cottage cheese or paté, with butter. Beverage or milk.

Notes
Live fresh yogurt or goat's milk is preferred to cow's milk. Where butter is mentioned, vegetable margarine may be substituted. If the dairy products are unacceptable, owing to catarrh or migraine or asthma, substitute soya milk, plant milk or other non-animal products. IT IS ADVISABLE TO AVOID THE USE OF SYNTHETIC SUGAR SUBSTITUTES.

Allowable Food and Drink
Vegetables
Asparagus, beets, broccoli, brussels, lettuce, mushrooms, nuts, cabbage, cauliflower, carrots, celery, sweetcorn, cucumber, beans, onions, peas, radishes, sauerkraut, tomatoes, turnips, swede, parsnips and any other vegetables not on the 'avoid' list.

Fruit
Apples, apricots, strawberries, raspberries, blackberries, grapefruit, melons, oranges, peaches, pears, pineapple, tangerines. May be cooked or raw with or without cream, but *without* sugar. *Never* have more than one piece of fruit at a time (e.g. one apple, one orange, etc.).

Juice
Any unsweetened fruit or vegetable juice, except grape juice or prune juice. *Avoid* tinned fruit juice unless pure.

Beverages
Decaffeinated coffee or herb teas.

Desserts
Fruit – fresh, stewed or baked.

Salt
Use sea salt in moderation.

Avoid Absolutely
Any foods not mentioned on the diet and, in particular: *sugar*; chocolate and other sweets etc., such as cake, pie, pastries, sweet custards, puddings, ice cream; salted nuts; and *all cereal products*; tinned foods; diabetic foods; syrup; molasses; and honey. Avoid ordinary coffee; tea, alcohol; soft drinks; beverages containing caffeine; tobacco; potatoes; rice; grapes; raisins; plums; figs; dates; bananas; avocados; spaghetti, macaroni and noodles. THESE DIETS SHOULD ONLY BE USED UNDER THE DIRECT AND REGULAR SUPERVISION OF A PRACTITIONER.

Why the Hypoglycaemic Diet?
When the majority of patients first encounter the diet prescribed for hypoglycaemia, they are understandably baffled by the ban on sugar. They have been given a diagnosis of low blood sugar and yet they must avoid sugar. Hypolgycaemia is the opposite of diabetes, and diabetics cannot have sugar; therefore, surely the hypoglycaemic sufferer must eat lots of sugar?

Another area of misunderstanding is the question of sugar falling when we miss meals. It has been acknowledged for many years that controlled fasting can be eliminative and rejuvenating. 'Why', the low blood sugar patient asks, 'do I feel so ill with an overnight fast, when prolonged fasts are frequently recommended at health clinics?'

Throughout our lives we are instructed and persuaded that sugar gives us energy. Sugar, honey, glucose and molasses are names synonymous with vitality. The hypoglycaemic patient is exhausted and depressed. It can, therefore, be very confusing to be told that he will feel better if he avoids all foods and drinks that are traditionally thought to provide energy.

There are sound physiological reasons why sugar and refined carbohydrates must be avoided. Neat sugar is absorbed too quickly and the body reacts by discharging insulin into the blood. We know that hyperinsulinism is the central problem in reactive hypoglycaemia, and sugar aggravates and perpetuates this problem. Our digestive system needs a small amount of carbohydrate in order to efficiently break down and absorb proteins and fats. This, however, can be supplied by taking non-refined carbohydrates (e.g. wholewheat bread, wholemeal cereal and the starch content in fruit).

In the context of blood sugar balance, the colour of the sugar is irrelevant. Both brown and white sugar have the same disturbing effects. Honey's sweetness is derived chiefly from sucrose (white sugar) and molasses has similar effects. For this reason both items are barred from the diet.

Synthetic Sugar

This may be a useful point at which to mention synthetic sugars. Although, from the purely chemical viewpoint, they should not influence the insulin-glucose balance, there are two facts worth noting.

1. If one needs to follow a low blood sugar diet for several months, and possibly always avoid sweet foods, it makes dieting considerably easier if all forms of sweetness are avoided, including synthetic sweeteners (e.g. saccharine).

2. Carlton Fredericks[34] maintains that synthetic sweeteners trigger the pancreas into activity rather like a conditioned reflex. He points out that even the smell of food can stimulate the gall bladder into activity and many physical changes (e.g. allergies, migraine, etc.) can be triggered off by the smell and taste of food.

Frequency of Meals

An important characteristic of the hypolgycaemic diet is the need for frequent meals. As we know, the hypoglycaemic patient produces too much insulin in response to certain foods, and the blood sugar falls. The only way to avoid a severe drop in the blood sugar is to eat small meals at frequent intervals. Frequent snack meals of starch (e.g. sandwiches, cereal, etc.) would serve only to aggravate the problem, as all forms of carbohydrate are absorbed very quickly. Protein and fats are, however, slowly absorbed and the sensitive insulin apparatus is not triggered. Small regular meals consisting of protein or fats serve to stabilize the blood sugar, and sudden rises and falls in the glucose level are avoided.

This levelling off of the blood sugar throughout the day is extremely important, as it is the *speed* of elevation that triggers off the insulin response and not the *amount* of rise (e.g. an increase of 70mg to 110mg of sugar in the blood will produce as much pancreatic response as a rise from 170mg to 210mg). The drinks between meals prevent overeating as they serve to reduce the almost unbearable craving for food so characteristic of hypoglycaemia. The milk drinks have the job of 'topping up' between meals, for without them the blood sugar would drop and symptoms would develop.

Proteins

I find the concept of a high protein diet unacceptable and unnecessary, and prefer to talk in terms of a 'protein-spread diet. This means simply, normal protein consumption with plenty of variety in choice of protein sources, but to have the protein at least four times daily. As I have already said, proteins and fats are absorbed slowly and do not upset the insulin-glucose ratio.

Fat is recommended in the diet as it depresses pancreatic activity. It should be remembered, however, that this diet is a short-term corrective programme, and it may be unwise to consume the amount of fat recommended in the diet for long periods. This particularly applies to patients with a history of heart or circulation problems, or with a high level of fat in the blood. (It is usual, if a high cholesterol or triglyceride factor is suspected, to measure these with blood tests before placing the patient on the high fat diet.)

Night-time 'Fast'

The diet requires that the patient has an early breakfast and a late supper. Both these meals should include either fat or protein. This recommendation is made to reduce the hours one spends 'fasting' throughout the night. As has been discussed many times in preceding chapters, the blood sugar normally falls to a low level between the hours of 3 a.m. and 5 a.m. The early morning asthma attack, the onset of migraine, panic feelings and anxiety, night-time raids on the pantry, etc. are all expressions of this phenomenon. By reducing the hours between dinner and breakfast, there is a good chance that the early morning crisis can be averted. The majority of people eat their last meal around 7 p.m. and have breakfast at 7 a.m. This twelve-hour 'fast' is too long, and careful, regular eating throughout the day is pointless if a patient develops a hypoglycaemic episode every night.

I advise patients to eat a small protein supper prior to going to bed (10.30 p.m. to midnight) and to have a glass of milk on waking (6.30 a.m.-7.30 a.m.). If, in spite of this, the early morning symptoms persist, I have at times recommended that patients set their alarm to wake around 3 a.m. and have a small meal. This may be tedious, but, if the early morning symptoms can be suppressed for two to three weeks, it can be considered to be well worthwhile. After such a time the diet and other measures have usually normalized the insulin-glucose balance sufficiently to allow the patient to sleep through the night.

Prolonged Fasting

Patients often ask the question, 'If fasting aggravates low blood sugar, causing distressing symptoms, why is it that patients in health clinics can fast for three or four weeks and yet feel marvellous?' The answer to this is in two parts. Firstly, they do not feel 'marvellous' — at least not during the first two days. Patients undergoing a fluid-only fast almost certainly experience many symptoms of hypoglycaemia. These include headaches, irritability, nausea, dizziness and indigestion. (A true hypoglycaemic patient would, of course, experience more profound and sustained symptoms).

Secondly, prolonged fasting does not cause a severe, progressive fall in the blood sugar. This is prevented by the process known as 'endogenous catabolism' which simply means that the body breaks down and utilizes its own fat and protein reserves. Seale Harris[8] has observed that patients who were literally starving to death owing to various forms of cancer, showed no symptoms of hypolgycaemia, the average blood sugar of the patients tested being between 84mg and 90mg. This compensation process that occurs during fasting only begins to operate after the third or fourth day after the fast, hence the initial drop in blood sugar during the first 48 hours of the fast.

Tea, Coffee, Alcohol and Smoking

The question of coffee, tea and alcohol consumption and the smoking habit has been covered in Chapter 9. All these substances, directly or indirectly, contribute to the hypo-glycaemic condition and must, therefore, be eliminated from the diet. It is particularly important to avoid the above list during the first few weeks of the diet, when the insulin response is still very sensitive. Dr Abrahamson[17] tells of patients whose hypoglycaemia was controlled by the proper diet, but who had severe blood sugar reactions when they took as little as *one* cup of coffee. Many investigators have shown that exposure to a smoky atmosphere can be virtually as harmful as smoking. For this reason the hypoglycaemic patient should avoid restaurants, theatres, parties, etc., where the atmosphere is often smoky.

Excessive Exercise

Although not detailed in the diet sheet, it is important that the hypoglycaemic patient avoids excessive exercise which will deplete the blood sugar level. (Many sufferers develop symptoms after heavy exercise, particularly migraine.) It will be obvious that stress and stress-inducing circumstances should also be avoided. The vicious circle produced by low blood sugar and stress is described in Chapter 2.

Supplementary Treatment

The regulation of sugar metabolism involves various glands and organs, chiefly the thyroid, pituitary and adrenal glands, and the liver and pancreas. It, therefore, follows that anything contributing to a malfunction or deficiency in these organs must also be a causative factor in hypoglycaemia.

There are certain specific substances that play an important role in sugar metabolism. When these nutrients are over- or under-supplied, the organs and glands involved in sugar metabolism may become over- or under-active. These minerals and vitamins are usually prescribed in conjunction with the corrective diet to speed up the normal activity of the sugar-regulating mechanism, and to minimize some of the unpleasant symptoms suffered by the hypoglycaemic patient.

Minerals
Zinc
There is a close relationship between zinc and insulin. Workers have shown that zinc can delay the absorption of glucose, leading, in some cases, to reactive hypoglycaemia.[36][37] It is also involved in the regulation of insulin release.[38] The usual supplementary dose is 20-30mg.

Chromium
Although chromium is a trace element and present in very small amounts in our diet, it is nonetheless of considerable importance in hypoglycaemia. In 1955 it was identified as the so-called 'glucose tolerance factor', and a deficiency of this mineral has been shown to produce altered glucose tolerance. In 1968 it was observed that glucose tolerance tests showed improvement in elderly patients by the simple addition of chromium to their diet. An interesting bonus achieved by taking chromium is its effect on cholesterol control. Research has shown that chromium can produce a drop of around 14 per cent in the blood cholesterol when added in relatively small amounts to the diet.[39] A supplementary dosage of 2-5mg (as chromium acetate) is usually prescribed for hypoglycaemia.

Magnesium and Calcium
The value of calcium as a dietary supplement, with particular reference to arthritis, has been outlined in Chapter 7. It is readily available in combination with magnesium, and sold as a substance known as Dolomite. Deficiency of magnesium can lead to liver damage,[40] and it is, therefore, usually included in mineral supplements for hypoglycaemia.

Potassium
Large doses of potassium are of value to treating a diabetic patient who has 'hypo-ed' or when a hypoglycaemic patient experiences a low blood sugar episode, (with symptoms of

anxiety, palpitations, dizziness, cold sweating, etc.). 1g of soluble potassium chloride taken at this time very often quickly relieves the symptoms. The stress produced by hypoglycaemia causes large amounts of potassium to be lost in the urine, mainly owing to adrenal exhaustion. The potassium chloride quickly makes up this deficiency, raises the blood sugar level and reduces the hypoglycaemic symptoms.[42]

I find that a daily dose of 200mg of soluble potassium chloride is adequate with the 1g reserved for acute symptom reactions. (This emergency treatment is of particular benefit when dealing with nocturnal anxiety, and is safer and more effective than the usual medical prescription of glucose tablets or sedatives.)

Vitamins
Pantothenic Acid
Adrenal exhaustion and hypoglycaemia are very closely linked, the common factor being the frequent lack of panto-thenic acid in both conditions. Research has shown that even a slight deficiency of pantothenic acid leads to a decrease in adrenal efficiency[43] with a subsequent imbalance in the sugar metabolism. Deficiency in this B vitamin also affects the insulin-glucose balance, causing the blood sugar to fall very rapidly when insulin is given.[44] [45] As I have said, the speed of fall is of the utmost importance in hypoglycaemia.

The Vitamin B Family
It is normal to prescribe a good high potency vitamin B complex with hypoglycaemia. They are of value in many areas of metabolism, aiding vitality, assisting assimilation of fats, and to some extent reducing the harmful effects of stress on the different organs and tissues. The B vitamins also serve to normalize sugar metabolism. Vitamin B_6[48] and B_{12}[47] are of special value in helping the adrenal glands, pancreas and the liver to normalize.

Vitamin E
Dr Shute and his colleagues in Canada have shown for over 30 years, the unique role played by this vitamin on circulation and tissue repair. Vitamin E is of specific value in encouraging the uptake of glucose (as glycogen) in the muscles, thus improving the hypoglycaemic symptoms.[49]

Vitamin C
The vitamin C requirement is often high when the adrenal glands are overworked or exhausted.[50] This vitamin is also of value in normalizing insulin production.

Acupuncture
This ancient therapy is frequently useful in reducing the unpleasant symptoms of low blood sugar. Auricula Acupuncture (treating the ear points) is particularly beneficial. In addition to the use of acupuncture needling, some practitioners inject vitamins into the ear points to improve the adrenal efficiency and rebalance the overactive pancreas. (This therapy is referred to as aqua-puncture.)[46]

Supplement Recommendations
Although the vitamins and minerals prescribed for hypoglycaemia vary according to the patient's past and present health history, the usual recommendations are as follows. These to be taken daily:

— Vitamin C – 2g (in divided doses).
— Vitamin B – 2 capsules (a good, natural high-potency formula).
— Vitamin E – 200mg-3 capsules.
— Calcium pantothenate – 100mg or 1 capsule.
— Dolomite – 3 capsules.
— Potassium chloride – 200mg.
— Chelated multi-mineral – 2 capsules.

N.B.
1. The mineral formula is chelated (bound to protein to aid absorption) and *must* contain chromium and zinc.
2. Vitamin E is only prescribed in high doses if the blood pressure is normal.
3. Vitamin C should be taken in divided doses throughout the day.
4. Potassium is readily available at any chemist as soluble potassium chloride.
5. With selected patients higher doses of various substances are prescribed when indicated. This applies particularly to vitamin E, vitamin B_6, vitamin B_{12}, folic acid and potassium.

Conclusion

As you will begin to understand, the diagnosis and treatment of hypoglycaemia is not a simple matter. The symptoms may be a reflection of serious organic disease, (remember that reactive hypoglycaemia has been called the 'great imitator'). This book is not intended as a treat-yourself manual, and readers are advised to consult a medical or non-medical practitioner who is familiar with the six-hour glucose tolerance test, and understands the symptoms and treatment of hypoglycaemia. In addition to accurate diagnosis, the treatment needs monitoring, as no two hypoglycaemic patients are exactly alike. Individual reaction to the diet and other treatment can vary considerably. Many patients miss the energy provided by the previous high sugar diet and reassurance and guidance is often needed.

A word here about the need for 'repeat' testing. Very rarely do I request a second glucose tolerance test. The taking of neat glucose can cause considerable symptom aggravation to the hypoglycaemic patient, (particularly after several weeks on the correction diet). The gradual loss of tenderness over the pancreas, coupled with the improvement in symptoms, is usually considered sufficient confirmation that the low blood sugar is normalizing. Repeated testing may be justified as a research tool, but the clinical priority is to the patient. It is difficult to justify to the patient the potential flare-up of symptoms caused by a second G.T.T., unless evidence is provided to show it is necessary.

Follow-up Treatment

As I have explained, the diet as outlined earlier in the chapter is essentially a short-term treatment. Except in very severe or complicated cases, the diet is prescribed for eight to twelve weeks. After this time the progress is such that a follow-up programme is recommended. This involves a diet consisting of wholewheat bread and cereal, fruit, salads, vegetables and good quality proteins and fats. Emphasis is placed on fresh, unrefined foods, and the avoidance of excesses of any kind. There are however still a few 'don'ts' to follow:

1. Avoid sugar and sugar-rich foods.
2. Avoid caffeine-rich drinks and drugs.
3. Restrict alcohol consumption.

4. Avoid smoking.
5. *Always* have a protein breakfast.
6. Never have a starch-only meal (e.g. bread and cake, cereal and toast).
7. Do not miss meals, particularly important when fatigued or under stress.

There is no need for this type of diet to lead to food fanaticism. The occasional homemade wholemeal cake or biscuit, in the context of a protein meal, should not cause trouble, nor should a glass of dry wine with meals.

If a patient's symptoms gradually return, I advise them to go back on their original diet. With time, most patients learn to understand their own tolerance to starch and sugar and by trial and error find a diet that they are happy with.

The hypoglycaemic diet with its emphasis on low sugar, coffee, tobacco and alcohol is, in many ways, a healthy approach to eating. Often patients find that their whole family (whether hypoglycaemic or not) benefit by following the diet.

Many patients starting the diet are concerned at the possibility of putting on weight (the diet amounts to 2500-3000 calories daily); this fortunately does not seem to happen, indeed most patients actually lose weight. Those who are underweight, often put on weight. This is not surprising when one realizes that the diet consists of very little carbohydrate, and very little sodium (salt). There is, therefore, a tendency to become more streamlined (owing to fluid loss) without losing a great deal of weight. Fredericks[34] has called this phenomenon 'biochemical spot reducing'.

12
HYPOGLYCAEMIA
CASE HISTORIES

The case histories that follow serve to illustrate the diversity of symptoms caused either partially, or totally by hypoglycaemia. For the sake of brevity only the major symptoms are listed. Many lesser symptoms are usually evident, as discussed in Chapters 1 and 2, and these all contribute to the hypoglycaemic syndrome.

The treatment and monitoring of the hypoglycaemic patient can be difficult and frustrating; as the treatment success depends largely on the patients' willingness to closely follow a strict diet. If this co-operation is provided, the speed of progress is often very dramatic and rewarding, but the response to treatment varies considerably as no two patients are alike. The twenty cases discussed could each provide sufficient material for a full chapter; but space only permits a brief description of each patient.

Case 1

Name:	Mrs O.
Age:	69 years.
Condition:	Migraine, duration over 30 years. Frequency – every 10-20 days.
Family History:	Mother, headaches and arthritis.
Diet:	High starch diet. 6 coffees daily with 2 teaspoonsful of sugar in each.

6-hour G.T.T.	mg/100ml	Summary	
	70	Fasting:	70
	105	Lowest:	49
	49	Fall:	21
	50		
	51		
	64		
	57		

Comments: Typical chronic migraine. Rapid fall in G.T.T. with very slow recovery.

Treatment: Dietary advice and vitamin supplements, with osteopathic adjustments to the neck.

Progress: No nausea; only occasional headache on rising.

Case 2

Name: Mrs. M.

Age: 64 years.

Condition: Agoraphobia with headaches, fatigue and overweight. Duration six years.

Family History: Sister, asthmatic.

Diet: High sugar diet. Smokes 30 cigarettes daily.

6-hour G.T.T.	mg/100ml	Summary	
	72	Fasting:	72
	123	Lowest:	50
	63	Fall:	22
	50		
	53		
	66		
	68		

Comments: Typical blood sugar curve establishing reactive hypoglycaemia.

Treatment: Dietary advice, acupuncture, vitamin and mineral supplements.

Progress: Very slow progress after three months' treatment.

Case 3

Name:	Mrs C.
Age:	72 years.
Condition:	Migraine. Duration 68 years.
Family History:	Father, lifelong migraine sufferer.
Diet:	Low sugar diet with low protein content

6-hour G.T.T.

mg/100ml	Summary	
82	Fasting:	82
122	Lowest:	48
156	Fall:	34
122		
48		
74		
78		

Comments:	Mild dysinsulinism with typical sluggish insulin response followed by inappropriate fall in blood sugar from 122 to 48.
Treatment:	Dietary advice and osteopathy.
Progress:	Good, but condition recurs with dietary changes.

Case 4

Name:	Mrs F.
Age:	56 years.
Condition:	Migraine. Duration 20 years with fatigue and history of asthma.
Family History:	Mother, migraine. Daughter, asthma.
Diet:	Average diet. 10 cups of tea a day.

6-hour G.T.T.

mg/100ml	Summary	
77	Fasting:	77
154	Lowest:	43
158	Fall:	34
48		
43		
58		
69		

Comments:	Characteristic rapid fall in glucose after the second hour, confirming hypoglycaemia.

Treatment:	Dietary advice, vitamin supplements and acupuncture.
Progress:	Excellent. Condition completely resolved after three months. No return of symptoms.

Case 5

Name:	Mrs G.
Age:	58 years.
Condition:	Tachycardia with irregular heart beats and palpitations. Duration 7 years. Overweight. History of severe stress and migraines.
Family History:	None.
Diet:	Erratic mealtimes with snack meals and little protein.

6-hour G.T.T.

mg/100ml	Summary	
77	Fasting:	77
125	Lowest:	50
146	Fall:	27
104		
50		
50		
61		

Comments:	Dysinsulinism with delayed insulin secretion, followed by inappropriate insulin excess causing rapid glucose fall from 104 to 50 with resulting slow recovery.
Treatment:	Dietary advice, mineral and vitamin supplements and acupuncture.
Progress:	Initially excellent, followed by temporary relapse due to family stress. Progress since has been irregular.

Case 6

Name:	Mr B.
Age:	44 years.
Condition:	Anxiety depression. Duration 30 years.
Family History:	Mother, migraine. Sisters, history of depression. Overweight.

Diet: Erratic snack meals consisting principally
                            of sandwiches and cakes.

6-hour G.T.T.

mg/100ml	Summary
63	Fasting: 63
121	Lowest: 33
145	Fall: 30
35	
33	
47	
42	

Comments: Delayed insulin secretion followed by
                            dramatic fall in blood sugar with very
                            slow recovery.

Treatment: Dietary advice, mineral and vitamin
                            supplements and acupuncture.

Progress: Treatment recently commenced; progress
                            minimal.

Case 7

Name: Miss R.

Age: 17 years.

Condition: Allergic rhinitis with seasonal hay fever,
                            headaches and frequent infections.
                            Duration over 2 years.

Family History: None.

Diet: High starch diet including sandwiches,
                            cakes and frequent snacks.

6-hour G.T.T.

mg/100ml	Summary
69	Fasting: 69
52	Lowest: 34
56	Fall: 35
34	
53	
58	
64	

Comments: Very rapid peaking and fall of glucose
                            level (highest point probably missed in the
                            test) followed by typical flat fatigue curve.

Treatment: Dietary advice and vitamin supplements.

Progress: Marginal, due to inability of patient to
                            follow prescribed diet.

Case 8

Name:	Miss O.
Age:	12 years.
Condition:	Hay fever. Duration over 4 years, with sensitivity to various foods causing headaches, stomach pain and fainting. Exhaustion.
Family History:	Mother, migraine; father, hay fever and headaches.
Diet:	Good but avoiding dairy products and eggs.

6-hour G.T.T.

mg/100ml	Summary	
68	Fasting:	68
89	Lowest:	61
64	Fall:	7
65		
68		
61		
67		

Comments:	Moderately flat fatigue curve.
Treatment:	High protein diet, vitamin supplements, osteopathic treatment with acupuncture.
Progress:	Excellent, symptoms completely cleared and able to eat some dairy products after 5 months.

Case 9

Name:	Mr K.
Age:	18 years.
Condition:	Eczema and bronchial asthma since birth.
Family History:	Grandfather, asthmatic.
Diet:	Average diet including 5 coffees daily with 2 teaspoonsful of sugar in each. Smokes 12 cigarettes a day.

6-hour G.T.T.	mg/100ml	Summary
	55	Fasting: 55
	84	Lowest: 43
	62	Fall: 12
	43	
	53	
	55	
	55	

Comments: Combination of flat fatigue curve and reactive hypoglycaemia. Unusually low fasting level.

Treatment: Dietary advice, vitamin supplements and acupuncture.

Progress: Initially good, particularly with the eczema. Asthma has tendency to recur if the diet is not followed.

Case 10

Name: Mrs L.

Age: 47 years.

Condition: Epilepsy. Duration 25 years. Worsened recently with agoraphobia and exhaustion.

Family History: Sister, migraine.

Diet: Irregular or missed meals. Excessive coffee and tea.

6-hour G.T.T.	mg/100ml	Summary
	80	Fasting: 80
	100	Lowest: 65
	80	Fall: 15
	65	
	80	
	80	
	85	

Comments: Mild reactive hypoglycaemia, but sufficient to produce symptoms.

Treatment: Dietary advice. Vitamin supplements, mineral supplements and acupuncture.

Progress: Good. Fatigue improved within 2 weeks. Mild anxiety persists but no symptoms of epilepsy.

Case 11

Name:	Mrs V.
Age:	58 years.
Condition:	Migraine over a period of 22 years with severe nausea, attacks occurring 3-4 times weekly. Underweight.
Family History:	Sister, migraine.
Diet:	High-starch, low-protein diet with numerous snacks throughout the day.

6-hour G.T.T.

mg/100ml	Summary
100	Fasting: 100
185	Lowest: 70
150	Fall: 30
70	
90	
135	

(Test discontinued – patient started vomiting)

Comments:	Pre-diabetic curve followed by rapid glucose fall and over-swing at the end of the test – possibly due to adrenal over-compensation).
Treatment:	Dietary advice and vitamin supplements and acupuncture with osteopathic treatment.
Progress:	Excellent. Symptoms completely cleared within 3 weeks.

Case 12

Name:	Mrs G.
Age:	33 years.
Condition:	Anxiety neurosis, attacks occurring at night, with fatigue and vertigo. Duration over 5 years. Frequency, every 5-7 days.
Family History:	None.
Diet:	Average diet. 5 coffees daily.

6-hour G.T.T.	mg/100ml	Summary
	66	Fasting: 66
	79	Lowest: 45
	52	Fall: 21
	48	
	45	
	59	
	59	

Comments: Typical flat fatigue curve with reactive hypoglycaemia confirmed and a very slow recovery.

Treatment: Dietary advice, acupuncture and vitamin supplements.

Progress: Progress slow due to concurrent drug treatment.

Case 13

Name: Mrs V.

Age: 35 years.

Condition: Typical hypoglycaemic symptoms of depression, exhaustion and anxiety. Onset 6 years ago, with birth of first child.

Family History: Mother, migraine.

Diet: Sparse, with low protein.

6-hour G.T.T.	mg/100ml	Summary
	59	Fasting: 59
	113	Lowest: 59
	171	Fall: −
	200	
	150	
	64	
	59	

Comments: Pre-diabetic. Severely delayed insulin response with subsequent rapid fall due to insulin excess.

Treatment: Dietary advice, vitamin supplements and herbal remedies. Osteopathic and acupuncture treatment.

Progress: Very slow, due to inability to follow prescribed diet and domestic stress.

Case 14

Name:	Mrs S.
Age:	32 years.
Condition:	Severe headaches with blackouts, poor memory, nausea and fatigue. Duration over 3 months and worsening.
Family History:	Brother, migraine. One child with asthma.
Diet:	Average diet but 20 coffees daily, 20 cigarettes daily and high whisky intake.

6-hour G.T.T.

mg/100ml	Summary	
64	Fasting:	64
151	Lowest:	33
168	Fall:	31
50		
33		
44		
50		

Comments:	Severe hypoglycaemia following insulin delay. Very slow recovery.
Treatment:	Dietary advice and vitamin supplements. Osteopathic and acupuncture treatment.
Progress:	Good with some relapses complicated by concurrent drug therapy.

Case 15

Name:	Mrs E.
Age:	57 years.
Condition:	Fatigue, headaches, dizzy spells, poor memory, overweight. Duration over 3 years.
Family History:	Mother, migraine; son, asthma.
Diet:	Average.

6-hour G.T.T.

mg/100ml	Summary	
63	Fasting:	63
90	Lowest:	38
38	Fall:	25
51		
52		
59		
59		

Comments:	Mild fatigue curve with severe fall in glucose level and slow recovery.
Treatment:	Dietary advice, acupuncture, osteopathy and vitamin supplements.
Progress:	Erratic, complicated by domestic stress.

Case 16

Name:	Mrs P.
Age:	30 years.
Condition:	Multiple sclerosis for 6 years preceded by history of severe migraine.
Family History:	Mother, migraine; brother, asthma.
Diet:	High sugar-caffeine diet. Smokes 20 cigarettes daily.

6-hour G.T.T.

mg/100ml	Summary	
68	Fasting:	68
75	Lowest:	40
80	Fall:	28
55		
40		
65		
69		

Comments:	Flat curve associated with poor absorption and diagnosis of reactive hypoglycaemia.
Treatment:	Dietary advice, vitamin and other supplements. Acupuncture and osteopathic treatment.
Progress:	Minimal. Treatment discontinued.

Case 17

Name:	Mrs N.
Age:	25 years.
Condition:	Migraine. Duration 12 years with associated paraesthaesia, nausea, dizziness, palpitations and fatigue.
Family History:	None.
Diet:	Excessive sweet-eater. High sugar-caffeine diet with frequent snacks. Voracious appetite.

6-hour G.T.T.	mg/100ml	Summary
	66	Fasting: 66
	139	Lowest: 50
	136	Fall: 16
	50	
	61	
	64	
	66	

Comments: Delayed insulin response with subsequent hypoglycaemia.

Treatment: Dietary advice and vitamin supplements.

Progress: Excellent. Symptom-free within 10 days.

Case 18

Name: Mr R.

Age: 56 years.

Condition: Stomach pain with severe headaches. Duration 30 years. Symptoms daily.

Family History: Mother, asthmatic. Both children have similar stomach symptoms.

Diet: Average diet with moderately high caffeine and sugar intake.

6-hour G.T.T.	mg/100ml	Summary
	82	Fasting: 82
	113	Lowest: 47
	108	Fall: 35
	51	
	47	
	61	
	85	

Comments: Classic sugar curve for a diagnosis of reactive hypoglycaemia.

Treatment: Vitamin and mineral supplements and dietary advice.

Progress: Symptom-free within 3 months.

Case 19

Name: Mrs A.

Age: 26 years.

Condition: Hay fever with fatigue and headaches. Duration 8 years. Past history of migraine.

| Family History: | Brother, hay fever. |
| Diet: | Average, but meals erratic. |

6-hour G.T.T.

mg/100ml	Summary
82	Fasting: 82
137	Lowest: 48
82	Fall: 34
48	
67	
88	
78	

Comments:	Good example of hypoglycaemic curve.
Treatment:	Dietary advice and vitamin supplements, osteopathy and acupuncture.
Progress:	Condition completely cleared in 5 months.

Case 20

Name:	Mrs I.
Age:	52 years.
Condition:	Headaches, 2-3 weekly. Duration 40 years.
Family History:	Brother asthmatic. Two children both with headaches.
Diet:	High sugar-caffeine diet, i.e. most exclusively carbohydrate. Smokes 10 cigarettes daily.

6-hour G.T.T.

mg/100ml	Summary
49	Fasting: 49
59	Lowest: 24
41	Fall: 25
24	
43	
54	
64	

Comments:	Severe low blood sugar with poor absorption and flat fatigue curve.
Treatment:	Dietary advice and vitamin supplements.
Progress:	Excellent, symptom-free within 6 weeks.

GLOSSARY

Acetone
Substance found in urine in fasting. Released in excessive quantities in the urine and breath of uncontrolled diabetics.

Acidosis
Said to occur when the compensatory mechanisms of over-breathing and creation of very acid urine are 'stretched to the limit' and drowsiness or coma occur. Ketone substances are present in the blood.

Adrenal Glands
Paired glands, also called the suprarenal glands, located adjacent to the tip of each kidney.

Adrenal Cortex
Outer layer of the adrenal gland – secretes the steroid hormones including cortisone.

Adrenal Medulla
Central part of the adrenal gland – secretes adrenaline.

Adrenalin
Hormone produced by the adrenal glands to facilitate sudden physical activity in emergency. One effect of adrenalin is to increase blood sugar.

Aetiology
The causation of disease.

Allergen
Substance which causes tissue to become sensitive.

Atherosclerosis
Narrowing of blood vessels.

Aura
Sensation, auditory or visual, experiences by patient prior to epileptic or migraine attack.

Calorie
The amount of heat required to raise temperature of one gram of water by 1°C. The total amount of heat available from full combustion of food is: from carbohydrate 4.1 Kcal/g, from protein 4.3 Kcal/g, from fat 9.0 Kcal/g. N.B. in nutritional and metabolic studies the Kilo calorie is generally abbreviated to Calorie but written with a capital C to indicate that it is the larger unit.

Carbohydrate
Energy-producing compounds of carbon, oxygen and hydrogen; (starch, sugar, glucose etc.).

Citric Acid Cycle
See Krebs Cycle.

Cortisol
Substance similar to cortisone released by the adrenal glands; also called hydro-cortisone.

Cortisone
A carbohydrate/protein-regulating hormone, released by the adrenal glands.

Cranial Nerves
A group of twelve pairs of nerves connected with the brain. These include the optic, trigeminal and vagus nerves.

Dumping Syndrome
A condition due to gastric surgery, where the stomach contents rapidly empty, producing a sudden elevation of blood sugar.

Dysinsulinism
Term implying disturbance of normal insulin-production. May therefore result in a combination of high and low blood sugar, usually considered to be pre-diabetic.

E.E.G.
Electroencephalogram – a record of the electrical currents developed by the brain.

Endocrine
Means literally secreted internally, applied to substances produced and released into the blood, especially hormones.

Endogenous
Arising from or growing from within; or arising from causes within an organism.

Enzyme
Substances produced by the body, acting as a catalyst by increasing reactions of various substances.

Epinephrine
Term used in the U.S.A. for Adrenalin.

Fructose
Fruit sugar also called levulose, found in all sweet fruits.

Functional Hypoglycaemia
Hyperinsulinism. See **Reactive Hypoglycaemia.**

Growth Hormone
Substance that stimulates growth mainly secreted by pituitary gland, exerts direct effect on protein, carbohydrate and fat metabolism.

G.T.T.
Glucose Tolerance Test.

Glycogen
A polysaccharide, the main carbohydrate storage material in man, formed by and largely stored in the liver; also stored in muscle. Known also as 'animal starch'.

Haemophilia
Congenital tendency to haemorrhage, owing to impaired clotting ability. Occurs only in males.

Hidden Sugar
Sugar in foods, see Table 3 for examples.

Histamine
Substance found in the body, released after injury also concerned with the control of tissue permeability.

Histaminase
Substance produced by the liver, acts by inactivating histamine.

Hydro-Cortisone
See **Cortisol.**

'Hypo' Effect
Hypoglycaemia produced in the diabetic patient owing to excess insulin dosage.

Hypothesis
A supposition, assumed as a basis of reasoning.

Idiopathic
Self-originating, of unknown cause. Used to describe disease of spontaneous angina.

Insulin
Hormone released by the Islet glands of the pancreas to control the level of sugar in the blood.

Islets of Langerhans
Small glands in the pancreas producing insulin.

Ketogenic Diet
High fat/protein diet; prescribed to encourage weight loss through breakdown of body's fat reserves.

Ketones
Acetone and allied substances resulting from breakdown of fats.

Ketosis
See Acidosis.

Krebs Cycle
The final process or pathway whereby food is broken down, being converted to energy; carbon dioxide and water.

Lactose
Milk sugar: breaks down to galactose and glucose.

Molasses
Thick sweet syrup, residue remaining after crystalization of sugar. Contains sucrose, fructose, calcium, potassium and many B vitamins.

Monosaccharides
Simplest sugar, e.g. glucose.

Neuroglycopenia
Symptoms produced that develops as a result of reduction of glucose supply in nerve tissue.

Oedema
Abnormal amount of fluid in tissue; causing swelling and puffiness.

Pancreas
Gland situated left upper abdomen, secretes digestive enzymes and insulin (also known as sweetbreads).

Pellagra
Deficiency of vitamin B_3 (nicotinic acid) causing dementia, diarrhoea and dermatitis.

Pituitary Gland
Master gland situated in skull; produces substances that influence thyroid, adrenals, growth, gonads and fluid balance.

Phospholipid
Fat-containing phosphorus, e.g. lecithin.

Physiology
The study of processes that occur in living system.

Polysaccharide
Carbohydrates containing more than two basic single sugar units in their molecule, e.g. starch, glycogen.

Psychosomatic
Relating to both mind and body.

Reactive Hypoglycaemia
Hypoglycaemia due to body's over-reaction to sugar. Also called 'hyperinsulinism'.

Relative Hypoglycaemia
See Reactive Hypoglycaemia.

Renal Diabetes
Diabetes, thought to be dependent on defective kidney function.

Renal Threshold
Concentration of a substance in the blood at which it appears in the urine.

Rickets
Deficiency of calcium availability to bones, usually due to vitamin D deficiency.

Saccharine Disease
Term used by T.L. Cleeve to define conditions caused by the taking of refined starch and sugar, e.g. coronary disease, peptic ulcer, etc.

Scurvy
Vitamin C deficiency, symptoms include haemorrhage of gums and swelling of tissue.

Starch
Carbohydrates made up of a chain of monosaccharide sugars, i.e. polysaccharides.

Sucrose
Disaccharide (double sugar); the molecule contains two basic simple sugar units known as cane or beet sugar.

Thyroid Gland
Gland located anterior throat. Secretes thyroxine which controls metabolism, growth and development.

Thyrotoxicosis
Hyperthyroidism, condition caused by excess production of thyroxine; leading to weight loss, rapid heart, etc.

Thyroxine
See Thyroid Gland.

Trace Elements
Mineral substances, present in the body in minute amounts, necessary for good health, e.g. cobalt, manganese, etc.

Transient Hypoglycaemia
Temporary low blood sugar, usually due to exercise, fatigue or missed meals. Usually reversible.

Trigeminal Neuralgia
Facial pain usually confined to branches of the trigeminal
nerve (one of the cranial nerves).

Triglycerides
Stored body fat; derived from the diet or synthesized in the
liver.

Vagal
Pertaining to the vagus nerve.

Vagus Nerve
One of the twelve cranial nerves, influences digestion. This is
effected during migraine attacks.

Vaso-dilation
Dilation of blood vessels.

WHERE TO SEEK HELP

The 6-hour G.T.T. is not a standard hospital test. For this and
other reasons, most G.Ps are not familiar with the diagnosis
and treatment of reactive hypoglycaemia. Those who are, are
usually in the private sector of health care. Practitioners of
alternative medicine; naturopaths, herbalists, acupuncturists,
homoeopaths and osteopaths, etc., are more aware of hypoglycaemia and are therefore more likely to know which of their
colleagues use the G.T.T. on a regular basis. Very few
practitioners in Great Britain test their patients for hypoglycaemia
with the six-hour G.T.T. For further information and practitioners names write to the following:

1. The Secretary, The Basingstoke Clinic, 54/56 New Market
   Square, Basingstoke, Hants, OR

2. Hon. Secretary, R.S.N.T. (Research Society for Natural
   Therapeutics), 94 Banstead Road South, Sutton, Surrey,
   SM2 5LH.

125

REFERENCES

1. E.A. Graham and N.A. Womack, 'Surgery of Hypoglycaemia', *Pract. Med. Ser.*, 1933.
   — 'Application of Surgery to Hypoglycaemic State due to Islet Tumors of Pancreas and other Conditions', *Surg. Gynae and Obstec.*, 1933, pp. 728-742.
2. Seale Harris, 'The Diagnosis and Treatment of Hyperinsulinism', *Ann. Intern. Med.*, 10, 1936.
3. M. Fabrykant, *Metabolism*, Vol. 4, 1955.
4. D. Anthony, 'Personality Disorders and Reactive Hypoglycaemia', *Diabetes*, Vol. 22, 1973.
5. D. Anthony, 'Hypoglycaemia and Personality', *B.M.J.*, 20 April, 1974.
6. W.E. Beebe and O.W. Wendell, 'Preliminary Observations of Altered Carbohydrate Metabolism in Psychiatric Patients' in *Orthomolecular Psychiatry*, edited by Hawkins and Pauling (W.H. Freeman, 1973).
7. P.L. Meiers, 'Relative Hypoglycaemia in Schizophrenia' in *Orthomolecular Psychiatry*, edited by Hawkins and Pauling (W.H. Freeman, 1973).
8. Seale Harris, 'Hyperinsulinism and Dysinsulinism', *Journal American Medical Association*, Vol. 83, 1924.
9. John Yudkin, *Pure White and Deadly* (Davis-Poynter, 1972).
10. H.J. Roberts, *New England Journal of Medicine*, 268, 562, 1963.
11. James Wilkinson, *Daily Express*, 31 July 1968.
12. E.P. Joslin, *Diabetes Mellitus*, (Lea and Febiger, 1971).
13. H. Kaplan, *Annals of Allergy*, 21, 41, 1963.
14. Malcolm I.V. Jayson and Allan Dixon, *Rheumatism and Arthritis* (Pan Books, 1974).
15. Hans Selye, *The Stress of Life* (McGraw, 1978).

16. Roger Williams, *Nutrition Against Disease* (Bantam, 1973).
17. E.M. Abrahamson and A.W. Pezet, *Body Mind and Sugar* (Holt, Rinehart and Winston, 1951).
18. *National Health Interview Survey*, 1966/67, U.S. Dept. of Health, Education and Welfare.
19. E. Cheraskin and W.M. Ringsdorf, *Psychodietetics* (Bantam, 1976).
20. Dr R.C. Atkins and S.M. Linde, *Dr Atkins Super Energy Diet* (Corgi, 1979).
21. T.L. Cleave, *The Saccharine Disease* (Wright, Bristol, 1974).
22. Dr R Ahrens, *The American Journal of Clinical Nutrition*, Vol. 27, 1974.
23. Dr B. Sandler, *Homeostasis*, Autumn 1974.
24. Roger Williams, *Biochemical Individuality* (University of Texas Press, 1970).
25. L.D. Lewis et al, 'Cerebral Energy State in Insulin-Induced Hypoglycaemia Related to Blood Glucose and to E.E.G.', *Journal of Neuro-Chemistry*, Vol. 23, 1974.
26. L.D. Lewis et al, 'Changes in Carbohydrate Substances, Amino Acids and Ammonia in the Brain during Insulin-Induced Hypoglycaemia', *Journal of Neuro-Chemistry*, Vol. 23, 1974.
27. B.T. Burton, Heinz Handbook of Nutrition, (McGraw, 1976).
28. E. Cheraskin, 'Cancer Proneness Profile', *Geriatrics*, August 1969.
29. J.F. Greder, 'Anxiety and Caffeinism: A Diagnostic Dilemma', *American Journal of Psychiatry*, 131 (10), pp. 1089-92, Oct. 1974.
30. L.K. Altman, *New York Times*, 15 March, 1975.
31. D. Cairns, C.W. Deveney et al, 'Mechanism of Release of Gastrin by Insulin Hypoglycaemia', *Surgical Forum*, Vol. 25, 1974.
32. G. Feurle, R. Arnold et al, 'Rise in Serum Gastrin during Insulin Hypoglycaemia with and without Simultaneous Gastric Aspiration', *German Medicine*, Vol. 3, 1973.
33. T.L. Cleave, *The Peptic Ulcer* (Bristol, Wright, 1962).
34. C. Fredericks and H. Goodman, *Low Blood Sugar and You*, (Constellation International, 1969).
35. Paavo Airola, *How to Get Well* (Health Plus Publishers, 1974).
36. J. Quartermain, Report Roulett Inst. 24. 100, 1968.

37. H.H. Sandstead et al, *Zinc Metabolism* (Ed. A.S. Prasad), p. 304 (C.C. Thomas, Springfield).
38. I.J.T. Davies, *The Clinical Significance of the Essential Biological Metals* (Heinemann Med., 1972).
39. H.A. Schroder, *Journal of Nutrition*, Vol. 94, 1968b.
40. L.A. Maynard et al, *Journal of Nutrition*, Vol. 64, 1958.
41. D.H.P. Streeten et al, *Journal of Physiology*, Vol. 118, 1952.
42. E.S. Egeli et al, *American Heart Journal*, Vol. 95, 1960.
43. H.F. West, *The Lancet*, 2, 877, 1958.
44. B.H. Ershoff et al, *Journal of Nutrition*, Vol. 50, 1953.
45. R.E. Hodges et al, *Journal of Clinical Investigations*, Vol. 38, 1959.
46. W.H. Khoe, 'The Treatment of Functional Hypoglycaemia with Acupuncture and Diet', *American Journal of Acupuncture*, Vol. 3, No. 4, Oct/Dec 1975.
47. H.R.V. Arnstein and R.J. Wrighton (Eds), *The Cobalamins* – A Glaxo Symposium (Churchill Livingstone, 1970).
48. Adelle Davies, *Let's Get Well* (Allen and Unwin, 1966).
49. W.E. Shute, Complete Updated Vitamin E Book (Keats, 1975).
50. B.H. Ershoff, *Nut. Rev.*, Vol. 13, No. 33, 1955.

INDEX